SKIN DISEASES

SKIN DISEASES

JAN DE VRIES

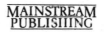

MAINSTREAM
PUBLISHING

EDINBURGH AND LONDON

First published in Great Britain in 1992 by
MAINSTREAM PUBLISHING COMPANY (EDINBURGH) LTD
7 Albany Street
Edinburgh EH1 3UG

ISBN 1 85158 453 6 (cloth)
ISBN 1 85158 454 4 (paper)

A catalogue record for this book is available from the British Library

Typeset in Palatino by CentraCet, Cambridge

Printed in Great Britain by Mackays of Chatham plc

Contents

Foreword

Jan de Vries, colleague and friend over many years, has dedicated his life to nature's medicine and to creating awareness of the benefits that it can bring to our health and well-being. His personal enthusiasm is an inspiration to colleagues and patients alike.

Jan's knowledge and experience as a natural health practitioner is communicated as always with an ease of style that is a joy to read. His book is a practical and common-sense approach to *Skin Diseases*.

As a sufferer of psoriasis myself for over 15 years, I remember well the feelings of discomfort, isolation and rejection that are associated with the disease.

My personal success with a holistic approach to healing the skin included careful attention to diet and used the resources that nature provided.

You too can have clear, healthy skin and new confidence in your life using this approach.

Jane Waters (Co-founder, Director)

The Alternative Centre for Psoriasis and Eczema Sufferers
The White House
Roxby Place
Fulham
London SW6 1RS

1

Skin Conditions

THE BODY is covered entirely with skin, from top to toe. This skin is in fact a very complex organ and has a totally different function than, for example, the skin of a cheese. A person's skin is responsible for many different functions. It is a mighty weapon, acting as a barrier against outside influences and has a vitally important role in maintaining a constant body temperature of 37 degrees Celsius. The skin also behaves like a third kidney, as in the control of perspiration: it filters out waste products and ensures that we do not dehydrate.

The skin is one of the biggest organs of the body and a man has roughly 1.5 square metres of skin, weighing about 4.5 kilogrammes with 10 kilogrammes of fat underneath. Contrary to the male, the skin of a female weighs about 3 kilogrammes and the fat underneath weighs 12 kilogrammes.

The skin is made up of two distinct layers. The outer or

superficial layer is called the epidermis, while the deeper layer is known as the dermis. During the first month of pregnancy, an embryo is covered by a single layer of ectodermal cells. During the second month the periderm develops over the surface. By the end of the fourth month, four distinct layers of skin are evident. The basal layer is known as the germinative layer and is responsible for producing new skin cells. This latter layer forms into ridges and hollows which we see as fingerprints on the surface. Fingerprints form the basis of many genetic studies and, of course, are used in criminal investigations. During the third and fourth months the lower layer is formed. This is the dermis, and the inner layer is called the subcorium, while the outer layer is known as the corium. The skin glands form in the corium and the deeper layer, or subcorium, consists of fatty tissue. The epidermis is responsible for the growth of nails and hair, and the dermis contains arteries and nerves.

Depending on what is required from the skin, it can be thick and rough, or fine and supple. Hormonal secretions determine whether the skin is dry or oily.

The cells of the epidermis house a substance called keratin. These cells are very thin fibres on the top layer of the skin. Keratin strengthens the skin and also makes it impossible for water to permeate, thus making us waterproof. There are also glands which ensure that water cannot penetrate the skin, and they secrete a fatty substance which destroys bacteria on the surface. This network which also consists of small blood vessels or capillaries in the cutis, penetrates the epidermis and carries nourishment to the follicles and the skin glands.

The elastic and collagen fibres which surround this structure do a highly efficient job. When we see how quickly the skin regenerates after a little damage, we realise that it deserves to be treated with great respect. It is really wonderful to see how a small cut is healed by so many invisible helpers. There are few tissues in the body that work as effectively as the skin and yet, on the whole, we take little care of this valuable, protective layer.

Keratin is a very important substance and is the main ingredient of nails and hair. Nails start to grow after two months' growth of the embryo in the uterus, and after five months the nails are fully developed. While the total thickness of the skin is only a few millimetres, finger nails grow at a rate of about one millimetre a week.

All over the body the skin is covered with sweat glands, with the exception of the lips. There are about three million sweat glands, mostly on the palms of the hands and the soles of the feet, and also the armpits. These allow perspiration to maintain the body temperature although, especially under the armpits, perspiration can often result in an unpleasant odour, and is also a common cause of many skin conditions. There are many deodorants available, although unfortunately a lot of them are of an inferior quality. Deodorants are available not only for use on the armpits, but also for other parts of the body. The deodorant should be chosen with great care. Those with an aluminium content are not very beneficial and nowadays special natural deodorants are available in health food shops.

Anti-perspirants are not such a good idea, as these block the sweat glands and prevent them from working normally. We can create a number of problems for ourselves by using the wrong products, and I have seen quite a few unidentified skin problems under the arms which have been self-inflicted. Care must be taken to select a good deodorant which has no side-effects. The same applies to deodorants for the feet. There are a lot of products which could aggravate or even cause a fungal skin condition and I have come across this on many occasions. In the case of sweaty feet it is much more sensible to sprinkle a little Borax powder into the shoes. This works extremely well and although it does not stop the feet perspiring, it will take away the odour.

It is worth remembering that blood circulation in the skin

is very important. The circulation of the blood is controlled by the hypothalamus, situated in the brain. This gland works like a thermostat in controlling the body temperature.

The outer horn layer of the skin contains the blood supply and different pigments, for example melanin, which determines skin colour, and sensory nerves. The sensory nerves in the skin are vital for our pleasure and protection. It is because of these nerve endings that we experience pain when we cut or burn ourselves, or pleasure when we are touched or stroked. It is also because of these receptors that we experience taste, itchiness or tickling. A healthy skin is of vital importance if we are to enjoy life to the full, and provided we take care of our skin it will look good all our lives. My mother, who was almost ninety when she died recently, still had a perfect skin. She always looked after it, and although she had a lot of tension, worry and emotional upset during her life, she maintained bodily cleanliness and a healthy spirit. A healthy skin was the visible evidence that her diet consisted of the right food.

It is said that, apart from the stomach, the skin is misused more than any other part of the body. Too often we are inclined to ignore the warning signs. Frequently we are careless when handling chemicals and often heedless of the contents of skin creams and cosmetics. Even so, the skin sends us all kinds of messages and warnings, sometimes in the form of an itch, while at other times warning signs are perceived in the form of a blister or rash.

Small itchy areas or skin rashes can be the start of major problems such as dermatitis or eczema. These problems can be caused, especially in young people, by incorrect eating habits. In a later chapter I will write in detail about such instances. However, it is broadly true to say that infantile eczema can be caused by an allergic reaction to various specific foods, and if this is not resolved, severe problems can result in later life. It is also essential to protect the skin when handling any sort of chemicals. Gloves must be worn, and care should be taken not to inhale any fumes. If a substance causes a reaction externally, it is easy to imagine what that substance might do to the lungs if it is inhaled.

Another source of skin irritation can be synthetic fabrics such as nylon and dralon. I have had to treat patients with some very nasty conditions because of allergies to these synthetic fabrics. Recently a charming young girl came into my surgery in the Netherlands with an extremely unpleasant, weeping, reddish skin condition. She was very upset and told me that she had been to doctors, specialists and faith healers, and every time the diagnosis was simply an 'unidentified skin disease'. I could see that she was desperate and her nervous system was stretched to its limits. She also told me that she had not been able to work for some time, and gradually her problems seemed to be getting worse. I talked for quite a while with her and it took some detective work to get to the root of the trouble: when I did some tests I found that hairspray, and the material used in some of her clothes, had triggered off this most unpleasant condition. She now has beautiful skin and is a much happier person. Too often people who suffer from skin conditions are told that they have to live with them, or that they are just unfortunate in having a poor skin.

I believe that every skin condition can be improved if it is treated correctly. A skin problem can be triggered off by something as insignificant as a hairnet, earrings or a small metal clip. Even the material used in the manufacture of our clothes can lead to skin problems. I need only look at my wife who, as a teacher, had the greatest difficulty in using chalk for writing on the blackboard, because, in her, it caused a skin reaction. Even a leather strap on her wrist-watch could trigger off an itchy condition. Very often minor details, seemingly insignificant, can be decisive in skin conditions. Skin problems may be so severe that people are unable to work, and yet the problem can often be cleared when the patient is desensitised. There are many methods in complementary or naturopathic medicine for dealing with such problems.

13

I remember a lady who consulted me about unusual swelling of the lips. No matter what she did, she could not overcome this. It turned out that it was her lipstick that was causing the problem but the more she tried to conceal the problem, the worse it became. The lips and nose can sometimes show the first signs of an allergic reaction to food, clothing, dust, pollen or in fact to anything with which we come into contact. With all allergies, the skin will soon let us know that something, somewhere, is out of sorts.

The skin provides excellent protection for the human body and reflects the state of our general health. I will always remember a patient, many years ago, who grew lettuces commercially. He lived in England, but was so desperate that he travelled all the way to my clinic in Scotland. He had a so-called 'unidentified skin problem' which was in an advanced state. The tests I carried out left me puzzled. I took blood tests and asked him what sort of chemicals, pesticides, fertilisers, etc. he used in his greenhouses. After a great deal of thought and testing, I came to the conclusion that he was allergic to the chemicals he used to obtain lettuces with an attractive green colour. I pointed out to him that not only was this chemical bad for him, but also for the customers who bought and ate this produce. Once I had discovered that he was allergic to this specific chemical colourant, it was easy to persuade him to grow his lettuces organically, which he now does. Colouring and preservatives in food can easily be responsible for triggering off many food allergies, which manifest themselves as skin problems.

With any skin problems it is very important that we look at our lifestyle and our habits. By a process of elimination we can often discover the cause.

Women are particularly vulnerable, because of their use of cosmetics. Real problems can be caused by using the wrong sort of make-up. Some eye shadows, or heavy creams, are especially likely to cause problems. I remember one case in particular, where a lipstick was taken off the market, because it was thought there was a danger of it causing a pre-

14

cancerous or cancerous condition. It pays to invest in a quality product, from a reputable skin care company. It is quite frightening to know of the many skin conditions which are caused by carcinogenic or questionable ingredients. It is not only the chimney sweep who comes in contact with soot, or the painter who uses creosote, who may be exposed to carcinogenic agents, but also the many people who work in the chemical and pharmaceutical industries. Certain chemicals may influence an existing carcinogenic condition.

It is important that we check up on the circulation of the skin and any other external signs. Especially with young children, it is easy to ignore a little irritation or rash. Yet, this is short-sighted as it could well be a fungus, which can spread rapidly in a relatively short time. Fungal problems are often ignored and yet they can be helped very effectively with some very simple remedies. It is not sufficient to treat these with a little cream or ointment, because by doing so we only manage to subdue the problem which will probably flare up again after a short time. Problems like these have to be cleared from the inside, and this is a point I will stress time and again in this book. Only by clearing the inside first will the outside skin condition be overcome.

When considering the development of skin conditions, it is important to note the psychological condition of the person concerned. Skin conditions can be triggered off by an emotional trauma. I have had quite a number of patients who developed nasty skin problems, for example shingles, after a time of constant worry, anger, or other psychological trauma. However difficult such conditions are to treat, they can be completely controlled with different herbal remedies. In such cases it is important for patients to help themselves by relaxing and trying to keep nervous conditions and stress under control. Often when teenage girls get a little spot, they become obsessed about it, producing an emotional reaction which is likely to result in a much greater skin problem. There is little point in trying to conceal spots under a layer of make-up, which often looks worse than the spot itself. In some cases medicines or drugs are prescribed to get rid of these spots, as it is a fact that an infectious skin disease may be caused by a bacillus. As I mentioned earlier, the condition of one's skin is a good indicator of one's general health, but the skin can also influence the functions of the heart, circulatory system, or the bowels, either negatively or positively. Too little sun can lead to a deficiency, particularly in vitamin D, while too much sun may lead to skin cancer.

Often we treat our skin unduly harshly and lack the intelligence or common sense warranted for such a delicate organ. Any sort of skin eruption deserves our attention. The easiest solution is often to take an antibiotic but this will make no impression on the root of the problem. Every skin condition is different and one has to identify the type of condition or eruption in order to be able to treat it properly. Consult a doctor or naturopathic practitioner who is experienced in treating skin problems. Whatever you do, never ignore it!

I was shocked recently when I heard about one of my favourite patients. I had treated this charming lady for many years, and I had grown very fond of her. When I returned from abroad a little while ago I was told that she had died suddenly from an unexpected infection. She was a great gardener and our love for gardening was something we had in common. While pruning her roses, she had scratched herself on a thorn. The skin reacted and an infection set in, which was so severe that it cost her her life. If action had been taken a little sooner, the story would probably have ended differently: any abrasion or wound must be taken care of immediately. This need not turn us into hypochondriacs or neurotics, it is merely a matter of common sense.

The skin is also a very important organ in the elimination process. Since the body of an adult contains over two million sweat glands, in order to achieve perfect health, every sweat gland must be in a condition to carry out its particular function. We eliminate the poisons from our body through the pores of our skin or sweat glands. If the glands are not active, there will be problems in the blood, the kidneys and the bowels. When these little glands are active, they excrete the harmful acids and waste material from our body. They also eliminate broken-down minerals and tissue. Two pieces of evidence point to a harmony between the sweat glands and other parts of the system. Firstly, when we perspire, the odour of dead gas is evident. Secondly, as proof of the elimination of dead tissue and decomposed minerals, you will find that when the sweat glands of the face become inactive, blackheads develop. If you squeeze these blackheads, on examination you will find a soft pasty substance. This is decomposed mineral and broken-down tissue, eliminated through the pores. Now, if this function is not performed properly and the body is not able to rid itself of these substances, but allows an accumulation in the sweat gland, a blackhead is formed, and all elimination through that gland is blocked. So, any waste products, including noxious gases, remain stuck within. When they reach the skin and are unable to escape, they condense into moisture which settles in different parts of the body, and starts decaying. This moisture, which can be called 'old water', weighs as much as 16 to 18lbs per gallon, while the specific gravity of fresh water is 8lbs per gallon. When the sweat glands fail to eliminate this refuse, it is taken into the lymphatic system, then into the bloodstream and must be carried to the bowel and filtered by the kidneys, in which case the kidneys would have to eliminate 16 times more than normal. This 'old water' begins to accumulate in the body and the flesh becomes hard and bloated. This in turn interferes with the sweat glands. There is less heat in the lower part of our body, because the circulation is less efficient further from the heart. Many people perspire freely from the forehead, palms of the hands and under the arms. This is because there is more heat in the upper part of the body. Perspiration is also noticed in the lower part of the body, as there are many sweat glands in this area which remain open and allow free flow from the inside, out through the pores. Perspiration odour in this part of the body can be strong, sometimes stronger than under the arms. The hair under the arms is supposed to keep the sweat glands free from blockage, so shaving the hair is unwise.

It is possible to locate problems in any of the organs of the body by paying strict attention to the skin. If there is a problem in the circulation, a cold patch will appear over the heart, whereas if the circulation is good, the entire chest will be warm. Lung or bronchial trouble may be detected by laying one's hand on the upper part of the chest, beneath the collar bone. Any difference in skin temperature can indicate a problem. If the problem is in the stomach or duodenum, one will find the cold spot on the front of the body underneath the diaphragm, just below the ribs. If the trouble is in the reproductive organs, one will find the cold spot just above the pelvic bone. With ovarian trouble, it seems to be nearer the hip bone. If there are problems in the rectum, such as piles, the cold spot will be found on the lower back, over the sacrum.

Every organ of the body will reflect its condition in signs on the skin. When there is trouble in the eyes, ears or throat, one will find cold spots on the head, the back of the neck, and the shoulders and arms. Over the location area of each organ there will be perspiration as the organ perspires. If, for any reason, the perspiration is checked, a cold spot develops: if the liver is not working properly, there will be a cold spot over the area of the liver as the action of the sweat glands is retarded. As the perspiration leaves the body in other areas, you will notice a particular odour, because of the retarded action of the liver. At times the odour of the body may be like that of the stomach and bowels, or like that of the kidneys after urinating. Feel for yourself by placing the palms of your hands on different areas of your skin.

The soles of the feet are also very important for elimination. Many people have caused themselves serious problems in the kidneys and the lower limbs because they prevent perspiration, using various solutions and patent medicines. As I said at the beginning of this chapter, it is terribly important that we do not prevent perspiration, just remove the odour.

There are a lot of skin conditions caused by fluctuating hormone levels, which dramatically affect the sensitivity of the skin. Especially in women, we often see that these particular problems become much worse before a period. We see this a lot with chronic skin conditions, and generally find that women who have problems with the ovaries, during their menstrual cycle also have problems with a spotty skin. Hormonal balance is therefore very important.

It is a mistake to think that men and women suffer from the same problems. Differences in hormonal condition mean that similar skin conditions in men and women have to be treated quite differently. The following example illustrates the difference between the skin of men and women. Take two people, one of each sex, and give them each a bar of soap and tell them to wash their hands in hot water until the hands appear spotless. Send the man into a separate room and allow him to touch nothing for three-quarters of an hour. The woman can continue with her ordinary routine, the only condition being that she does not touch soot or grease. If at the end of 45 minutes they both wash their hands again, the woman will leave no dirt in the water, whereas if the man just dips his hands in the water and then dries them on a towel, he will leave a dirty mark. This goes to show the differences in the skin of a man and a woman and it follows that diagnosis and treatment will need to be totally different.

Similarly, a young man with spots may worry about his spots preventing him being attractive to the opposite sex. However, they are not the same spots that a teenage girl with a similar skin condition would have. The hormone system can be greatly helped with some simple herbal remedies, which are effective for severe problems as well as milder conditions. It is important to look at the problem holistically, taking into account attitude, mental outlook, and all the physical signs and symptoms. There is no point in using lots of expensive creams and lotions. The problem ought to be treated internally, as well as by following the correct diet.

The ancient Greeks strived for harmony and balance within the body. This points to yet another approach to skin care which involves looking for causes of disharmony or chaos. Sometimes we treat our skin badly, without being aware of it, for example by following the wrong diet, smoking or drinking excessively. If the cause is not addressed, chaos will be allowed to spread throughout the body, disrupting the major organs, and disturbing the body's inner harmony. Many people will then start to treat the skin superficially and cover their spots with layers of make-up for camouflage. This will not provide a lasting solution. We must get to the root of the problem, look for the cause, and when the problem is solved the skin sufferer will feel a great deal happier.

There are far too many skin conditions to deal with all of them in this book. I have only mentioned some of the more common ones, and some of those skin conditions I have treated over the many years I have been in practice. I am sure that all skin conditions can be helped. Once the practitioner has diagnosed the condition, he can advise the patient on how to treat his or her particular problem, and mostly I favour a naturopathic treatment, which in my experience is extremely effective. The body's self-healing powers can be greatly assisted with proper care of the skin and by maintaining the body functions in good order. Mother Nature takes good care of her children, as long as we obey her simple laws.

2

Eczema

ECZEMATOUS DERMATITIS is a skin disease which can be acute or chronic and is characterised by erythema, papules and vesicles with varying degrees of inflammation, crusting, scaling and skin eruptions. Usually this term is used for eczema in general and of all the different kinds of eczema, this is probably the most common, and certainly not to be underestimated. This frequently chronic skin condition, marked by an ugly rash, can be a plague, not only for teenagers, but also for adults. Unfortunately it is impossible to say that one particular treatment will help each and every sufferer. From experience I have learned that each case is different. There may be a thousand patients with the same type of eczema, but each and every case must be judged individually and the treatment varies according to the circumstances. For some patients the eruption may be controlled quickly, while in others it may be of a persistent nature. Certain patients may react to heat, while the condition in others will flare up as a result of cold. However, both sexes are subject to the same annoying irritations, such as itching, which is always present and which usually becomes more troublesome at night. Burning or smarting is another frequent complaint. The acute form, often characterised by oedema or crusting and oozing, is capable of causing lesions everywhere, much to the patient's annoyance and embarrassment.

Not an easy problem, and yet it can be controlled. If the patient is willing to co-operate, this eczema, which can be hereditary or may be caused by an allergy, can be cleared. Once the cause has been diagnosed, treatment can start, but in general it is very important that dietary management is revised.

It may help to know that each square inch of human skin, which is about five square centimetres, contains 20 million cells. Cell renewal is necessary, especially with persistent skin problems such as this kind of eczema. A healthy diet is essential to encourage cell renewal. Any food allergy problem is capable of prolonging the condition for a considerable period of time, even if the best treatment is applied, as it could spoil the whole programme. If there is an allergy problem, anything from the pig, for example pork sausages, bacon, ham or gammon, should be avoided, as well as white sugar, white flour, spices, alcohol and chocolate. Liberal amounts of fruit and vegetables, and lots of mineral water or even distilled water should be taken. Be very careful with any colourings or additives.

One ought to be aware that correct nutrition goes far beyond the art of selecting the right food and that over-nutrition can be as big a problem as malnutrition. Time and again an almost immediate improvement will be seen when dairy products are omitted from the diet, as these tend to aggravate eczema. Non-citrus drinks are important and it is essential that an abundance of fruit and vegetables, and even their juices, must form the major part of our diet. Nothing can take the place of a piece of fruit, and it is the life force within these living foods that often allows for improvement or cure of even the most chronic conditions. Food must play a major part and in this context I must point out that of equal importance is the knowledge that germs thrive on junk food.

Besides milk, eggs are another frequent source of food intolerance. Some eczema sufferers react almost immediately after eating an egg and its high protein content can easily trigger problems, even in a controlled and stabilised situation. In my book *Nature's Gift of Food*, there is much more information on this subject and in dietary recommendations I never allow more than three or four eggs a week. In some cases of eczema, eggs may need to be totally eliminated.

Wheat can also cause major problems. In many lectures and publications I have emphasised that wheat, because of artificial processing of the grain, can cause unidentified skin diseases. Wheat, which once may have been considered a superior nutritional source for mankind, has almost become an enemy. Nowadays the most surprising results may be obtained when an eczema patient is prepared to take my advice and change to a completely wheat-free diet. There are plenty of substitutes for wheat and people with persistently chronic eczema are advised to replace wheat with buckwheat, millet, potato flour, rye, rice or soya flour. Wheat is used in many more food items than might be expected and it does pay to read the labels carefully. There are so many products on the supermarket shelves which contain wheat, that at times this may be rather confusing, but will certainly be worthwhile.

It is surprising to see how many people's diets have deficiencies and I dare say that most eczema sufferers are deficient in essential fatty acids. The daily diet is lacking in so much nowadays, that it is not unusual to detect a deficiency at the root of quite a number of health problems. In many such instances it is sensible to use oil of evening primrose, as it is a rich source of essential fatty acids. A series of double-blind, placebo-controlled studies in the

Department of Dermatology at the University of Bristol, involving both adults and infants with atopic eczema, demonstrated a great improvement after the use of oil of evening primrose. In the analysis of the blood samples, the improvement was ascribed to the gammalinolenic acid (GLA). The rich source of linoleic acid in evening primrose ensures that three weeks of oral treatment can bring about significant improvement. The reports on this trial were fascinating and the 'before and after' effects with adults and children were carefully recorded.

It may be that you have not heard of evening primrose. I have mentioned this substance in quite a few of my books, and I was one of the very first practitioners in Great Britain who prescribed this food supplement as a remedy, with great results. Until recently evening primrose was unknown in the West and yet it is a healing herb which has been used by the native Americans for at least five hundred years. It is a wildflower which grows along the eastern seaboard of the United States and Canada, and it is thought that it may have originated in Central or South America.

Essential fatty acids cannot be manufactured by the body and can only be gained from food. There are several theories about essential fatty acids, but it is clear that, like vitamins, linoleic acid has no biological activity on its own. Unless linoleic acid can be converted to gammalinolenic acid, it has no activity as an essential fatty acid (EFA). EFAs are very important for several reasons. They are the constituents of cell membranes in the cell tissue of the body and play a vital role in determining the biological properties of those membranes. A high level of gammalinolenic acid is the precursor for prostaglandins, a significant factor in the control of many biological functions. GLA production in humans can be affected by many factors, such as saturated fats, sugar and alcohol, and is therefore a useful dietary supplement.

I have already mentioned that EFAs are a vital part of the structure of all cells, not least of which are those of the skin. EFAs help to strengthen the membranes of the cells and the tiny blood vessels called capillaries, and prevent an increase in skin permeability, and also moisture loss. EFAs also assist in maintaining a hormonal balance, which is very important, and will help in the regulation of functions such as the digestive and absorption systems. So often eczema and psoriasis sufferers experience problems of excess acidity. There are many theories regarding the 36 acids in the human body, and the explanations of mineral and acid behaviour are very closely linked. Therefore I often advise the use of certain minerals or mineral salts.

The three essential gases, oxygen, nitrogen and hydrogen, are naturally penetrating gases, freely absorbed by the lungs. When combined, these gases help to produce the moisture for lung expansion. The minerals, passing into the body, change their disposition and colour contact. The natural way of transmitting minerals through the human body is different for every individual and the slightest deviations in bodily conditions can cause radical changes. In fact, a sluggish lymphatic system can be the reason for a complete disharmony in these areas. Taking mineral salts of sulphur can greatly assist the absorption process. The water or moisture that is passed through the tissues looks like pink acid. When, by the natural force of flow, the acid created by the yellow salt of sulphur comes into contact with the acid of the alimentary canal or red part of the body, a change takes place, allowing the two acids to create a third acid of an entirely different disposition. Each mineral produces an acid of the same colour, and when combined with others, a new acid is created. Thus the various acids are multiplied again and again until the necessary acids have been pro-duced and distributed throughout the different parts of the body. On hearing about the 36 acids of the human body, it may be surprising to learn that there are yet many more acids that are actually detrimental to the human system. A certain percentage of acid is necessary to carry out the daily functions of the human body and these are the acids that are mentioned most frequently.

We also have acids, created by dead gases in the system, that are dangerous and detrimental if they are allowed to remain in the body. There is a complicated scientific reason for this, but it is good enough to know that as long as the body has a sufficient quantity of various minerals, equally balanced in the acid condition, it will take care of itself. When a mineral enters the body it is as a moist, transferred gas and each one has its own identity in the form of wave patterns. When a mineral contacts the mineral of its own vibration, in a certain organ, it immediately takes on the natural colour of that organ. As the tissue of the organ absorbs the gas, it becomes a solid mineral, forcing out the dead or decomposed mineral, creating new life and new activity in the organ. The dead mineral is then forced into the channels of elimination and so, out of the body, provided the circulation and elimination systems of the body are working normally. If this is not the case, you will find proof of the action of the minerals, either in an uncomfortable feeling in the bladder, gallbladder or kidneys, or in the formation of stones in these organs. You may now understand why I stipulate that any signs of acidity in the body deserve immediate attention.

When there is over-acidity, which I notice often in urine samples of eczema patients, every method possible should be used to restore the balance. One of the best ways to do this is to use the remedy Centaurium in combination with sulphur. In mineral form, sulphur is a constituent of the amino acids, hormones, vitamins, sulphates and enzymes in the oxidation-reduction process where it forms several links. It is essential for good skin, nails and hair, and purifies the system. Sulphur is an essential element of the human body as it plays an important role in the acid-based balance and fortunately there are a considerable number of natural food sources that contain sulphur, for example vegetables such as kale, onions, turnip, cauliflower, beans, brussels sprouts, and chives.

Earlier I mentioned the suitability of Centaurium in combination with sulphur. Centaurium is a herbal preparation for digestive irregularities and lack of appetite, from the Bioforce range and, combined with sulphur, it plays an important role in the acid-alkaline system. Moreover, it has anti-allergenic properties especially useful when a wheat allergy is suspected. It is marvellous to know that the Creator of mankind has even made provision for the many allergic manifestations that nowadays occur with respect to wheat. Centaurium – largely composed of a cornflower extract – is an excellent remedy, not only as an anti-acid, but also for digestive problems caused by wheat. It also serves to reduce inflammation.

Dependent upon the circumstances, I sometimes also recommend taking some Urticalcin together with the Sulphur-Centaurium combination mentioned above. Urticalcin also belongs to the Bioforce range of remedies, and is a homoeopathic calcium preparation consisting of a few calcium compounds and stinging nettle. In this combination it forms a balanced and easily absorbed calcium, which is so important for eczema problems. It strengthens the bones and is also excellent for brittle nails, loss of hair and skin complications.

It is always beneficial to take a complete vitamin, mineral and trace element supplement. In this respect I can wholeheartedly recommend Health Insurance Plus from Nature's Best, which I consider one of the best and which I have prescribed for years. Taking just one tablet daily will usually be sufficient. It provides a broad-based supplement to safeguard one's health. The latest research has gone into this product which explains why so many practitioners are prescribing it, and why so many people use it as a protection, even more than a cure. This multi-purpose formula offers a broad spectrum of recognised essential nutrients, and in its hypo-allergenic base it is guaranteed to be free of wheat, grains, soya, corn, yeast, artificial colours, preservatives, flavourings, and common allergens, including salicylates and dairy products. This explains why I often prescribe it for people who struggle with eczema problems.

The Bioforce range has another herbal remedy that is unparalleled for skin problems. The base for this remedy is the pansy or viola, hence the name given to it by Dr Vogel, Violaforce. This fresh herb preparation, especially effective for cradle cap and all kinds of eczema, is a specific therapy for all skin rashes, in young and old.

This leads me to another form of eczema which is, as the name suggests, predominantly found in babies and young children – *Infantile eczema*. Nowadays we hear about it much more often and it can indeed be an extremely unpleasant problem. Often infantile eczema is caused when the mother, who feeds the baby on breast milk, suddenly has to stop for whatever reason, and the baby is weaned and given cow's milk instead. Frequently the digestive system of small children is unable to cope with the high protein content of cow's milk which provides nine times more protein than mother's milk. Mostly this is the background to infantile eczema, which sometimes even leads to an asthmatic congestion problem. Quite often mothers themselves recognise the problem and enquire if the baby or toddler will suffer from a lack of calcium if they are taken off cow's milk. I can reassure them that soya or goat's milk is very often preferred at such a young age when one has to be especially careful not to create problems for the future, which may develop into far worse conditions than skin trouble or asthma. Urticalcin, the homoeopathic calcium tablets mentioned earlier, will erase any doubt of a calcium deficiency. A simple remedy like Violaforce is often the answer for the immediate problem at hand and the sooner these little ones are helped, the better.

Another problem which contributes to the misery of eczema in both adults and children is caused by the nervous system. This may well become somewhat erratic as a result of skin irritations and, in turn, demand extra attention. There is a distinction between the voluntary nervous system, which we control consciously, and the involuntary nervous system, over which we have no conscious control. The latter is constantly in action and is controlled by the heart, while influencing various functions of the body. A third division of nerves, occupying the skin and part of the flesh of the body, influences certain portions of the lymphatic system. These groups of nerves are so interwoven that they interconnect with each other in various parts of the body, each group having a connection with the brain.

The voluntary nervous system is controlled from the objective part of the brain, and it controls muscle action as in the neck, turning the head, and the movement of the arms and lower limbs. There are many muscles in our body that are consciously controlled. The winking of an eye, opening and closing the mouth, the movement of the tongue, the voluntary muscle action in the anus and the muscles of the bladder, are normally subject to our will. With eczema problems, either in adults or infants, we often see that it is on these parts of the body where the eczema is most active. It is also there that an osteopath can effect some little adjustment in order to control the voluntary nervous system a little better.

The sympathetic nervous system is the preferred name for the involuntary nervous system, as its action never ceases. It is constantly operating throughout the organism. The sympathetic nervous system branches out between the third and fourth bone in the neck. I have sometimes been referred to as the 'third cervical practitioner', as I have often had to make adjustments to this vertebra. I must stress that this adjustment may only be done by a fully qualified practitioner. The third cervical vertebra controls the whole sympathetic nervous system.

Dietary management is also important for eczema sufferers, as the stomach, with the aid of the sympathetic nervous system, creates the continuous motion of the lining of the stomach, causing the food to move slowly, mixing it with gastric juices, which is the first step in digestion. Food is formed into small ball-shaped pieces which travel downward into the duodenum, where bile from the liver and secretions from the pancreas and gall bladder mix. The rotary motion of the sympathetic nervous system also extends down through the small intestines to the colon which looks like a corrugated tube. When the food material enters the ascending colon, these corrugations, aided by a form of gas, elevate it to the transverse colon. Then the rotary motion of the sympathetic nervous system carries it on to its destination, and eventually out of the body.

In the lower part of the body we find a large group or mass of nerves, called the sacral plexus, just above the lower end of the spine. Attached to the short ribs, commonly known as the lumbars, is a large nerve extending down to the sacral plexus, and at this plexus or nerve centre, the three nervous systems connect. The voluntary nerves continue down the spine to the sacrum, where a group of four voluntary nerves leave the spine and connect with the sacral plexus. The nerves of the skin also connect with the sacral plexus, from the lower part of the stomach cavity. The sympathetic nervous system connects to this plexus and extends from this nerve centre to every organ in the lower part of the body. It extends from the eyes down, through the interior organs, to the sacral plexus and down to the anus, connecting with both creative and urinary organs, and with the rectum. Much of the nerve energy of the lower limbs and feet is also controlled from this centre. There is another important group of nerves that extend down the spinal column from the base of the skull to the coccyx. This group is known as the sympathetic trunk and is held in place by a fibrous tissue that connects with the vertebrae of the spine. The sympathetic trunk connects with the voluntary nervous system and is connected by other nerves to the sacral plexus.

The three nervous systems are very complicated. From different sections of the spine, groups of nerves control the actions of different parts of the body. The second lumbar plexus controls the flexion of the hips, and the third has much to do with the action of the knees. The first, second and third joints in the coccyx control the muscles of the legs and the movements of the feet. The last joint of the spine or coccyx controls the skin from the base of the spine to the anus. The third section of nerves, the nerves of the skin, leaves the spinal column at the base of the skull and is controlled by the subconscious, or that portion of the brain located in the lower part of the back of the head. The sacral nerves appear to be the contributory nerves from the voluntary system. They supply the flesh of the lower limbs, and extend upwards through the muscles of the lumbar region and have a great influence on the sacral plexus.

The reason for explaining the workings of the nervous system in some detail, is to demonstrate the close connections between the skin and the nervous system. The itchiness associated with eczema and infantile eczema can cause loss of sleep for which I prescribe 10 drops of Dormeasan. This is a safe herbal remedy for restful sleep that can also be given to very young children. Dormeasan is a combination of *Melissa* (balm), *Avena sativa* (oats), *Passiflora incarnata* (passion flower), *Humulus lupulus* (hops), and *Valeriana and Lupulinum* (hop grains). This fresh herb preparation for mild sleep disorders and stress, has a calming effect when over-excited or restless. It is also beneficial for nervous exhaustion as well as mental over-exertion. It is of great help in such conditions and, when taken in combination with some other remedies, it has helped to clear many a case of infantile eczema.

For the almost incurable eczema and psoriasis sufferers who have really been through all the channels of doctors, dermatologists and hospitals, without any long-term or lasting effects, I always advise making a fresh start. However, before starting on any alternative medication it is wise to give the body a total cleanse, and the best way of achieving this is by using the Rasayana Cleansing programme, or the 'Spring Cleaning Course'. In India this cleansing programme is sometimes called a 'Rasayana Kalpa', or Life Extension programme.

In the ancient medical system of India we find what is one of the oldest and most time-tested approaches to medicine, herbal treatment, nutrition, and health. Ayurvedic (Science of Life) medicine comprises a body of medical tradition that extends back at least several thousand years. Through its long history, Ayurvedic medicine has incorporated a wide range of different therapies. These range from herbal medicine to physical therapy and massage, surgery, psychiatry, the use of medication and many other treatment modalities. As a result, the school of Ayurvedic medicine has a breadth and depth that is possibly unparalleled in the history of medical science. This has made it possible for Ayurvedic physicians to develop an extremely complex and complete science of herbology (botanical medicine). Long before we discovered their use in the West, traditional Hindu physicians were using herbs to lower blood pressure, calm nerves and regulate the rhythm of the heart. They were even using fungal preparations, similar to penicillin, as antibiotics. Their practice of surgery was very advanced for the time. As far back as twelve hundred years ago there are accounts of successful surgery, such as the replacement of ears and noses that had been severed in battle.

The old Hindu physicians did not treat just the disease, but treated the sick person as a whole. One of the best things that we can do for our body as a whole is to cleanse and detoxify it internally. When we begin to feel sluggish and unable to do things as well as we used to, or do not feel as good as we did in the past, it may be time to clean up the system and get it on the right track again.

The following five herbal formulae serve to perform a thorough cleansing, regulating and rejuvenating programme. The glands in the body that produce external secretions are stimulated so strongly that during the first three days some loose bowel movements may occur. The functioning of the liver, gallbladder and bile duct will also be strongly stimulated. The kidneys will receive a thorough cleansing and be stimulated and regulated. With a strong

32

emphasis on good nutrition during this programme, not only will digestion improve, but also the inter-relationship between the liver, kidneys, gallbladder, intestines and stomach will be returned to a more natural state.

Herbs for Ten to Fourteen Days Cleansing Programme

Arabiaforce

Function: Stimulates proper digestion of food and tones the stomach and intestinal tract.
Useful for motion sickness.

Dose: 10 to 15 drops in a small amount of water, apple juice or rosehip tea – morning and evening.

Contents: Aloe, cola nut, Peruvian bark, bitter orange, sweet myrtle, yellow gentian, myrrh, frankincense.

Comments: This herbal formula affects the stomach by regulating and calming the stomach nerves. This in turn creates the ideal conditions for proper digestion. Due to its effect on the stomach nerves it is also an excellent remedy for the prevention of nausea and motion sickness.

Rasayana 1

Function: Blood cleanser and purifier. Stimulates function of intestines. As a laxative it stimulates elimination without becoming habit forming. This combination also acts as a mild diuretic.

Dose: Two tablets twice daily (morning and evening) with Arabiaforce.

Contents: Senna leaves, buckthorn bark, aloe, uva ursi, fennel, chicory, blessed thistle, fumitory, dwarf elder, rest harrow, wild ginger, elecampane

Comments: This formula affects the functioning of the

glands in the intestines and can be used in place of harmful laxatives. Due to the stronger secretion of the glands, functioning of the intestines is stimulated. Should stronger stimulation be indicated, take three to four tablets, which will be sufficient for most cases. For children it is generally enough to crush one tablet and give it to the child mixed with juice or cereal. This formula is not habit forming and after it has been taken for a period of time, it brings lasting results as long as sensible nutritional habits are maintained.

Rasayana 2

Functions: Stimulates liver and gallbladder. Increases secretion of bile in cases of liver dysfunction.

Dose: Three to five tablets with a glass of water after lunch.

Contents: Indian saffron, aloe, centaury, dandelion root, quickgrass, sarsaparilla, barberry, St John's wort, club moss.

Comments: This herbal formula has a soothing as well as a stimulating effect on the liver and gallbladder. Since the secretions of bile will increase, it is of utmost importance to first take care of the proper functioning of the intestines (using Rasayana 1). In cases of chronic or stubborn constipation, it is recommended that one does not begin taking Rasayana 2 until proper bowel function is achieved.

Nephrosolid

Functions: Stimulates kidney and bladder function. Useful for kidney and bladder problems and increased urinary discharge.

Dose: Take five to ten drops in a small amount of

water three times daily with some Golden Grass Tea.

Contents: Golden rod (European), silverweed, birch, rest harrow, wild pansy, knotweed, horsetail, juniper.

Golden Grass Tea

Functions: Stimulates kidney function, urinary discharge and acts as a mild disinfectant.

Dose: Pour one pint of boiling water over one heaped tablespoonful of tea. Allow to steep for 10–15 minutes. Drink some throughout the day.

Contents: Golden rod (European), birch leaves, knotgrass, horsetail, wild pansy.

Comments: Under the programme described here, many toxic substances are eliminated through the kidneys. It is advisable to support, regulate and cleanse the kidneys because of this. This is best done by sipping small amounts of the Golden Grass tea throughout the day. This formula should never be boiled, but rather should be steeped slowly. The tea can be taken either cold or warm, but without sugar. If you must sweeten it, use honey. It is very important that this tea is taken a little at a time, perhaps a sip every 15–20 minutes. If you are working or travelling, just keep a cup or flask nearby. When this tea is taken over a period of time, it will have a generally strengthening and stimulating effect. When combined with Nephrosolid and the other three formulae, the body will experience a feeling of renewed strength and well-being. The person who follows a cleansing course once or twice a year, will experience a general improvement in health, and eliminate many substances that might otherwise seriously affect the health.

The various formulae in this programme not only cleanse and regulate, but also help to make the different organs work in a more harmonious relationship with one another. Individuals suffering from serious constipation problems should undergo two or three programmes until all is regulated, rejuvenated and functioning well. It is very important to take these formulae at the advised times and in the recommended sequence. Therefore, pay particular attention to the directions given under each herbal formula heading. For this programme to be effective, it should be followed for at least 10–14 days and may be continued for up to three weeks.

This particular programme will give the body a good foundation that can be followed with many kinds of treatment. Never give up! The most challenging exercise is to cure what is thought incurable. Give it your undivided attention, keep fighting and you will win.

3

Dermatitis

THE LADY who sat opposite me in my consulting rooms
would have been considered extremely attractive, but her
skin detracted from her beauty. She told me about frequent
spells of improvement, always followed by periods of deterioration. I felt utterly frustrated, although recognising that
it was even worse for her, because there was absolutely no
lasting improvement in her condition, despite all my efforts.
This lady suffered from a long-standing condition of *Contact
dermatitis.* She had an acute superficial inflammation of the
skin, which I was sure was caused by an irritant of either
animal or mineral origin. Often the cause of such a condition
is to be found in the home or at work. There are also a
number of plants, such as ivy, chrysanthemum and
especially primula, which can bring on dermatitis. Sometimes fruits or vegetables, or chemicals, can be the cause,
and certain patients can gradually become extremely sensitive to a certain plant or herb. Nowadays it is important not

to overlook the possibility of hair dyes, hair lacquers, certain face creams or lipsticks initiating or aggravating a skin condition. Clothing material too, can be a causative factor and it was the latter that was the culprit with this particular lady. Eventually I discovered that she had several outfits made of a certain synthetic material. Once this factor had been eliminated, there was a definite improvement.

What was nearly as bad as the actual skin inflammation was that, because of the length of time she had suffered from this condition, her immune system had also deteriorated. Quite often I am asked if I am serious when I claim that immunity plays a part in such conditions, and I definitely am. The same applies to allergies which very often disappear when one concentrates on the rebuilding and strengthening of the immune system.

For this lady I prescribed three remedies, which eventually cured the problem. A healthy immune system is able to deal with viruses, bacteria and toxins before they have a chance to become established. The world today is full of challenges to our defence mechanism. Some of these are under our control, such as the food we eat and the stresses and strains of work, but others are not. The latter include environmental pollution by potentially toxic chemicals. In these circumstances it makes sense to protect the integrity of our immune system by safeguarding our nutrition. I am a great believer in the supplement called Imuno-Strength, made by Nature's Best, which is a special formula that incorporates herbal remedies such as Devil's Claw and Echinacea. The combination of vitamins and herbal ingredients has made this a most popular supplement, and this eventually helped to cure this lady's condition.

I also treated this lady for an unhealthy bowel movement. It is very important with all skin complaints that the bowel function is regular and that the flora in the bowel is healthy. Healthy bowel bacteria must be allowed to flourish. These are sometimes referred to as 'friendly bacteria' and quite rightly so, as they are essential to a well-functioning system.

A healthy bowel flora is important as constipation ought never to be tolerated, most especially not by people who are troubled with skin conditions. Under these circumstances the digestive and bowel function should work absolutely efficiently. With certain skin conditions an active *Candida albicans* is sometimes recognised, which is a yeast parasite, and then I am likely to prescribe *Acidophilus* or *Lactobacillus*. If there is chronic constipation, it is advisable to use Linoforce. This remedy has been carefully researched by Dr Vogel and I am sure that its success is due to its two main ingredients – flaxseed and senna leaves. It is equally successful for either occasional or chronic constipation, as Linoforce increases the frequency of bowel movement. It also helps to regulate intestinal activity and forms the motion as it should be, which is a soft jelly mass. Chewing half a teaspoon of these grains twice a day will effectively deal with any constipation problems.

Finally, large doses of Echinaforce should be used. This is a natural antibiotic, but also a great healer for skin conditions. I mostly prescribe it for skin complaints, because, as a general antiseptic, it is most helpful. Dr Vogel decided to use both herb and root of the *Echinacea purpurea* for this remedy, which has proved to be an ideal combination. In many cases I have seen better results obtained with this remedy than with chemical antibiotics. This fresh herb preparation works as a non-specific stimulant therapy and it increases the body's own resistance, in the case of inflammations and infections, reduces susceptibility to infections, and is a great preventative for colds and flu. Taken internally, it helps many dermatological problems, often even in septic processes like carbuncles, abscesses or skin inflammation. Echinaforce is a great healer and I prescribed this also for the lady I mentioned at the beginning of the chapter. In her case I increased the recommended dose to 30 drops – three times daily. The results were more than justified.

Echinacea Cream is for external use only, but has similar properties to the remedy to which its name is so closely

39

related. It is a herbal skin cream made from the fresh herb extract of *Echinacea*, plus wild pansy extract. These extracts are combined in a moisturising base to produce a cream that is absorbed quickly and readily into the skin. This allows the active ingredients in the herb extracts to begin working immediately without leaving an oily residue. It soothes, moisturises, relaxes and protects the skin and may be used on reddened, irritated skin, or for minor wounds. It is also suitable for use under make-up or wherever moisturising is desirable.

Although I did not prescribe Seven Herb Cream for this lady, I feel that this is too good an opportunity not to mention another cream in the Bioforce range. This cream contains seven different herb extracts which are combined with avocado oil, lanolin and other oils, as well as beeswax. Due to this lubricating basis, Seven Herb Cream soothes, softens and nourishes the skin while promoting healing. This cream is recommended for use on poorly nourished, dry or rough skin and nappy rash. It is also suitable for cracked or fissured, badly chapped skin or lips, flaking skin, use after shaving, and on raw areas of the nose irritated by colds, hay fever, etc.

I used the knowledge I had gained in the treatment of the lady in question on yet another patient, a lady with a condition known as *Neuro dermatitis*, sometimes also called *Lichen simplex*. This chronic superficial inflammation of the skin, which had produced thickened, dry, demarcated plaques of an irregular oval shape, had associated itself with a severe pruritus. It was a most painful and troublesome condition and the poor lady had suffered much and sought help from every direction, all to no avail. As her facial skin was badly affected, she understandably felt very embarrassed, and, although she was a well-balanced person, it had nevertheless affected her nervous system. I felt very sorry for her and tried to help her with all kinds of methods, from diet to remedies. I was able to help her somewhat, but was not successful in finding a complete cure for her problem. Neuro dermatitis is a difficult condition to clear and I have had to look to contacts elsewhere in the world to find a possible solution. When I looked into some products from Japan and saw the results of a remedy called Shiso Perilla, an extract from the shiso plant, I found an answer for this patient. Again, my philosophy that nature provides an answer for every illness was confirmed, if only we look in the right direction.

This did not seem too easy with a young man I once treated for an eruption of the skin and the mucous membranes. His condition was called *Dermatitis medicamentosa*. Certain drugs can cause this condition and the eruptions from which he suffered were quite bad. He was a very tense type of person and that indicated that I also had to use some homoeopathic remedies to help him in this respect. It was clear that his condition had developed mainly because of the drugs he had taken and because of certain allergies from which he suffered.

Many skin conditions have their origin in a vitamin deficiency, especially a shortage of vitamins B and E, and because this young man's condition had become chronic, I had to use some special herbal and homoeopathic remedies. I used Symphosan, containing *Symphytum officinalis*, witch hazel St John's wort, Golden Rod, Sanicle, Houseleek and *Arnica montana*, and that combination was of great help. I also advised that he should refrain from using coffee, tea or chocolate, and suggested a substitute coffee, e.g. Bambu. However, I discovered that because of his condition, he suffered from severe stress and emotional problems, and therefore I prescribed Stress B-Vite, a supplement from Healthcrafts. His stressed condition was certainly a detrimental influence on his skin problems and I suspected that he was on the verge of a nervous breakdown. Stress had made him allergic to heat, noise and pollution, and he had lost much of his self-esteem. All factors that aggravated his condition. A simple stress test, put together by two American psychologists, shows the levels of stress caused by different events:

EVENT	STRESS SCORE
Death of spouse	100
Divorce	73
Marital separation	65
Personal injury	53
Marriage	50
Being fired	47
Retirement	45
Sexual problems	39
High mortgage	31
Child leaving home	29

From the above chart we can see that the stress score reflects the amount of change each life event generates. The greater the change, the higher the level of stress. Even joyful events, such as getting married, can be highly stressful, and are quite likely to cause a dormant skin condition to flare up.

This young man, because of the tranquillisers he had taken to reduce stress, had lost a lot of the benefit from the vitamins, minerals and trace elements in the prescribed supplements. No wonder the skin, which is the outward sign of our inner health, showed that there was a problem. Action was essential, not only dietary, but also in the form of supplements and help in reducing stress. A healthier lifestyle, and the ability to relax should help to restore most, if not all, of those overspent units, but if the pattern does not change, then one should not expect to see great improvements.

Some of the more common symptoms of stress are as follows:

PHYSICAL
Feeling tired much of the time
Disturbed sleep
Loss of appetite or craving for
  sweet things

EMOTIONAL/MENTAL
Easily irritated
Depression
Nightmares

Rapid heart rate	Moody
Restless	Unable to concentrate
Upset stomach	Anxiety/panic attacks
Weepy	Indecisive

The patient with the Dermatitis medicamentosa problem went from a severe depression into a decline with his personal relationships, developed feelings of acute embarrassment, and was often totally exhausted. He increased his smoking and drinking, which of course only made things worse.

Stress, one of the major problems in this day and age, weakens the immune system, increases the risk of illness, and further lowers resistance to stress itself. In all skin problems where stress is a factor, it is wise to take extra nutrients, such as: the B Complex group of vitamins (which include Thiamin (B_1), Riboflavin (B_2), Pantothenic Acid, Pyridoxine (B_6), Folic Acid, and seven other vitamins) are vital allies in combating stress and depression.

The B Complex group is responsible for mental health, a healthy nervous system, efficient digestion and a clear skin. Our need for B vitamins increases with the amount of stress in our lives. B vitamins are water soluble and cannot be stored by the body. There is a greater likelihood of deficiencies occurring within this group than with any of the other vitamins: it has been estimated that up to 70 per cent of the population in Europe and the United States of America suffer such deficiencies, as a result of the refining of grains and sugar.

As much as two-thirds of our daily calories are provided by foods which have been largely, or entirely, stripped of their natural B vitamins. While some of these are replaced by the manufacturers, such 'enrichment' replaces only a small part of what has been removed. Frozen meat can also lose much of its B vitamin content in the water and blood which escapes during thawing. Our ability to make our own B vitamins is impaired by antibiotics, so remember to increase your intake of B vitamins if your doctor prescribes a course of antibiotics.

This group of vitamins is further depleted by taking sleeping pills, smoking, alcohol or use of the contraceptive pill. It is essential therefore to ensure that the diet contains plenty of foods rich in B Complex vitamins: wheatflakes, muesli, porridge oats, wholemeal bread and biscuits, cottage or other cheeses, eggs, bananas, nuts and raisins, meat, liver, green vegetables, pulses, beans, rice, and dried fruit. A B Complex supplement can prove helpful, especially if you are under a great deal of stress or unable to eat a balanced diet that contains an adequate supply of B Complex vitamins.

Working alongside the B Complex vitamins, vitamin C is essential in the production of anti-stress hormones. Without adequate supplies, the body is unable to convert normal hormones into these stress beaters. Also a water soluble vitamin, it is easily destroyed by modern food processing and needs to be replaced or replenished daily. Levels of vitamin C are also depleted by smoking, alcohol, the contraceptive pill and stress. Vitamin E, a fat soluble vitamin, is found in the oil from nuts, seeds and grains. As well as maintaining healthy blood vessels, vitamin E protects the body's nervous system – vital at a time of stress. Specially formulated stress supplements such as Healthcrafts' Stress B-Vite are available, providing a balanced formulation of B Complex vitamins, vitamin C and a range of nutrients which help the body to cope with the pressures and strains of modern living.

The young man in question started to use Stress B-Vite on my recommendation and he was also more than willing to make certain changes in his diet. He was anxious to reduce his stress and fortunately accepted and heeded my advice. The manufacturers of Stress B-Vite have spent much time and effort on research into stress, and their findings are very interesting. They have produced a programme called

'The Stress Busters' and, in combination with Stress B-Vite, this has been well received. The programme is as follows:

Stress Busters: Eight Ways to Peak Performance

If things start getting on top of you, follow the stress management steps described below to reduce your stress to a level which is comfortable for you.

1. Try to adopt a philosophical attitude towards life's ups and downs. Learn to look on setbacks as valuable learning experiences rather than a reflection of personal inadequacy. Practise remaining cool, calm and collected in the face of setbacks and frustrations.
2. Try to avoid being drawn into too many battles on the part of others, since this depletes your own ability to resist stress. Never feel guilty if, despite your best efforts, you sometimes cannot avoid letting people down. Don't take remarks made in the heat of the moment too personally, or believe that it is a disaster if not everybody you meet likes you.
3. Learn to say no, politely but firmly, whenever unfair advantage is being taken of your good nature.
4. Avoid investing all your energy and enthusiasm in any one activity or task, especially if this is not fully appreciated by those you work for, or with. Develop a variety of interests. Pace yourself so that you don't run out of energy and simply abandon an idea. Organise life so that there are always plenty of new things happening, with various projects at different stages of development.
5. Keep a stress diary in which you note situations, people or challenges which make great demands on your stress reserves. Jot down what happened, who was present, how you behaved and what you thought. Rate the incident according to the number of Stress Resistance Units (out of 100) you feel were used up. Such a record makes it easier to identify RED zones in the week: times of day, people, places or events most likely to trigger a

45

stressful response. Now try to find ways of reducing or avoiding those situations.

6. Safeguard your health by taking regular exercise and watching your diet. Exercise, such as brisk walking, cycling, jogging or vigorous swimming, helps reduce stress and promotes a positive attitude. Work sufficiently hard to raise your pulse rate, but never so strenuously that it becomes impossible to hold a conversation through breathlessness. Provided you are able to talk comfortably, the level of exercise is about right.

   Eat fresh fruit and vegetables and avoid too much food high in carbohydrates, but low in vitamins – such as sweets. Complement your vitamin intake with a specially formulated stress supplement, such as Stress B-Vite.

7. Carry out the following relaxation method twice daily – ideally first thing in the morning and last thing at night. Take the phone off the hook and if necessary hang a 'Do Not Disturb' sign on the door. Find a quiet room, put on some soothing music, and sit or lie down, so that you are comfortable. Remove your shoes and loosen any tight clothing. Start by tightening up all your muscles as follows: clench your fists; try to press the back of your wrists against your shoulders; hunch your shoulders; clench your teeth; press the tip of your tongue to the roof of the mouth, and frown hard. Push your head back against the chair or bed.

   Take a deep breath, flatten the stomach, squeeze the buttocks together, stretch the legs and point the toes. Hold this tension for a slow count of five.

   Now let go. Allow the muscles to flop. Notice the difference between tension and relaxation in the muscles. Keep the breathing light and, each time you inhale, feel more tension flowing from the body which is growing warmer and heavier.

8. After relaxing the body, unwind the mind by picturing a pleasant, relaxing scene, such as lying on a sun-

warmed beach or in a beautiful garden. Notice the smell of the sea, or flowers, the warm sun on the face. Spend five minutes there, before returning to the real world.

Finally, it would be unfair not to mention the benefits of vitamin E for skin problems. Not only in the case of the young man, but in all skin conditions, vitamin E is extremely useful and complementary to any other remedy. Vitamin E – Alpha Tocopherol – is the most powerful vitamin of the body's anti-oxidant defence system. It is also the prime agent that prevents fatty acids from reacting with oxygen to form harmful toxins, known as lipid peroxides. Not only does vitamin E protect fats in the body, but other vital nutrients such as vitamin A, B Complex vitamins and vitamin C are also protected. Anti-oxidant vitamin E allows a more efficient use of oxygen by the blood and muscles, so it is favoured by sports people, working to increase their stamina and endurance, by training the heart and circulation.

Vitamin E is also necessary for the health of the reproductive system, the integrity of red blood cells, and for the functioning of the vital cells of the immune system. I find that Nature's Best Alpha Tocopherol is 36 per cent more potent than other supplements and I particularly like the fact that it is derived entirely from soya beans, which in themselves are beneficial to the skin.

Scientists from a New York university performed a study on the healing effects of vitamin E. The stability of skin grafts was very much improved by a vitamin E supplement and even in patients with deep vein thrombosis, a remarkable improvement was recorded. Because vitamin E is a fat-soluble anti-oxidant, it is able to protect against lipoperoxidation. There are many ways that vitamin E can be administered to treat all skin conditions, including the many different kinds of dermatitis. Each one needs an individual approach in order to be successful.

4

Acne

FACING ME was an attractive young woman. It was her misfortune that she was one of the many people troubled with *Acne vulgaris*, a condition which is very difficult to control. She was particularly upset because her wedding day was not far off and the stressful situation, extra work and sleepless nights were making her condition worse. It seemed like a vicious circle, because the more she worried, the worse her acne became, which in turn made her worry still more. During my many years in practice I have often come across similar situations and I cannot help but sympathise: I know that compared to other serious health conditions acne can be viewed as a trivial complaint, but this doesn't alter the fact that the sufferer is often emotionally insecure. More so, as this affliction often rears its head during the sensitive years of teenagers, which are so important in their mental development. Whether it concerns teenagers or adults, acne vulgaris can be a tenacious problem. If it is treated in a sensible and intelligent manner, much distress can be avoided.

What is acne vulgaris? *Merck's Manual*, the physician's handbook, says that it is a common chronic inflammatory disease of the sebaceous glands and the pilosebaceous follicles of the skin, characterised by papules, pustules, cysts, inflammatory plaque or nodules, and usually associated with seborrhoea. It is said that the exact cause of acne vulgaris is unknown, but that there are predisposing causes, such as an increased activity of the pilosebaceous complexities and very often a hormonal imbalance, which is why teenagers in particular have so many problems. Hereditary influences can play a role and certain foods have been known to aggravate this problem. A good rule to remember is that a healthy diet is important. There might also be some infection, like staphylococcus and possibly allergies play a role. In other cases there are deficiencies of vitamins, minerals and trace elements, and problems of sudden flare-ups caused by the digestive system.

In women, the ovaries play a large part, and this is often the reason why before, during or after menstruation, acne sufferers experience sudden flare-ups. If there is a real problem, and it is allowed to run on unchecked, the condition may well continue until the age of thirty or so. In most cases, however, if the patient co-operates, I have been able to control the condition to a large extent. Hygiene is essential and thorough cleansing is necessary. It is most important that the patient co-operates and does not pick or squeeze, which can cause lesions and permanent scarring, and it is certainly no use covering the spots with a layer of make-up. If this is considered necessary, it helps to be discriminating in the make and amounts used. Hydrotherapy treatment can often be of help, especially if an ioniser is used, and ultraviolet treatment may also be beneficial. Natural sunshine is best, but in our northern climate it may be necessary to supplement this with ultraviolet rays.

I reassured the bride-to-be that her skin would improve

greatly if she followed my advice and I emphasised that she was not alone in her plight. Some 70–75 per cent of all teenagers get acne. The hormonal change in teenagers is substantial. The hormones act on the thousands of small glands in the skin, and if the skin produces too much sebum, the chances are high that acne will develop. When blocked, the glandular ducts and pores form blackheads. Infection, combined with swelling, is the cause of the problem, and when the skin is not thoroughly cleansed, it becomes very rough and sometimes very dry or greasy. Washing certainly does not help to overcome acne, it just keeps the surface clear of excessive grease. It is much better to care for the skin with a cleansing milk or a very mild soap. It is also important to be aware of excessive perspiration, as this too can aggravate an acne condition. I must stress that squeezing, pushing or rubbing the spot is to be discouraged, as the fragile skin is easily damaged and scarred.

Many sufferers enquire hopefully if their acne will ever disappear completely. It certainly does disappear but the timing varies: in some cases it may take a long time, whereas with other people it will disappear quickly. Although predominantly a teenage problem, acne can cause a number of conditions from early childhood to adulthood, affecting both male and female. A young man from Belgium recently visited my clinic in the Netherlands. After hearing his story I realised that he had become very introverted as a result of his skin problems. He was very keen to find a girlfriend, but his acne had given him an inferiority complex. I told him that his acne problem could be cleared, but suggested that in the meantime he might consider growing a beard. He admitted that he had never thought of that and was certainly going to give it a try.

Even the most effective treatment will take some time, especially if the condition has been allowed to persist. Acne problems may take time to respond to treatment, but eventually they will be overcome. I always see a great improvement when Echinaforce is used, as it increases the body's own

resistance to inflammation and infection. Inflammation processes are reduced and quick healing is to be expected when
this remedy is used. Many a time I have heard patients
comment appreciatively on how soft and smooth their skin
has become after using Echinaforce. This natural antibiotic
kills the bacteria in the spot and dries the surface of the skin.
Even when the skin is very greasy or very dry, it harmonises
and conditions the skin, and therefore I have no hesitation
in recommending this herbal preparation for acne vulgaris.

For unusually persistent conditions I also prescribe
Petasan, because this remedy promotes quick healing.
Petasan is a combination of *Viscum album* and *Petasites
officinalis*, commonly known as Butterbur, and it is ideal for
any nutritional deficiencies, as well as acting to make the
skin supple. If the skin problems are related to the monthly
cycle in women, and the skin condition deteriorates during
specific times of the month, the homoeopathic remedies
Ovarium D3 and Sepia D6 are extremely helpful. These
stimulate the ovarian function, so balancing monthly menstruation. Sepia will help the yellow spots on the face and
will take away the inflammation of the ovaries, any skin
rash, excessive perspiration, and warts. An excellent combination for an acne vulgaris problem.

It is also important to take some extra vitamins and
vitamin E in particular is essential. I find Nature's Best
vitamin E products excellent, because of their considerable
anti-oxidant properties. I have already explained that vitamin E is a fat soluble vitamin, occurring naturally as substances called tocopherols, four of which provide vitamin E
activity in the body. Of these, alpha tocopherol is the most
potent, providing the greatest nutritional and biological
activity.

It is important that you choose your supplements with
care. Laboratory tests have shown that some vitamin E
supplements contain low potencies with poor vitamin E
activity. Nature's Best have taken great care to provide a
selection of different vitamin E formulae, derived from

100 per cent pure soya beans and carefully researched to guarantee the highest quality. The anti-oxidant properties of vitamin E ensure protection to body cells and tissues, which helps to maintain the health of the skin, muscles, red blood cells, fatty tissues and pituitary gland. Increased polyunsaturated oils and fats in the diet will cause increased oxidation of vitamin E, so adequate supplies must be available from the diet.

As an informed health enthusiast, it is important that you should know whether your alpha tocopherol supplement originates from nature or from a chemist's test tube. Why? Because weight for weight, the active alpha tocopherol derived from natural sources is 36 per cent more potent than the synthetic alpha tocopherol. Nature's Best provide only one vitamin E product containing the dL form. The innovative Hypo E capsules are produced to meet the demands of those wishing a guaranteed, good value, hypoallergenic formula. The rest of the range contains only the natural D alpha tocopherol.

To obtain faster results, vitamins A and D should be taken together. Vitamin A, which is often called the skin vitamin, will help you obtain a better, younger looking skin, as well as healthy hair and nails. Without these vitamins the skin would soon die and begin to appear rough. Nature's Best provides vitamin A either as preformed vitamin A or as Carotene, both of which are found naturally. This fat soluble vitamin is required for the growth and repair of almost every body tissue. Also a powerful anti-oxidant, it is required for night vision and for the development of teeth in young children. Nature's Best Vitamin D Plus A combination is another excellent product. Involved in the uptake and regulation of calcium and phosphorus from the intestinal tract, vitamin D is required for healthy bones and teeth. Nature's Best uses only the natural form – vitamin D3 or cholecalciferol. Two potencies are available: vitamin A 5000 IU plus vitamin D 400 IU, or vitamin A 7500 IU plus vitamin D 400 IU.

For all kinds of acne and skin problems the use of oil of evening primrose is beneficial, and I will talk about this product in more detail later. Adele Davies, who was one of America's leading nutritionists, hit the nail on the head when she stated that essential fatty acids were very necessary. What Adele Davies did not know was that my great-grandmother had already realised the vital force present in evening primrose. I might be accused of repeating myself, because in most of my books I have sung the praises of evening primrose, but this is because I know its value for keeping certain problems under control, both inside the body and externally. Why is evening primrose so necessary in treating cases of acne vulgaris? Evening primrose has been considered a healing herb for many centuries, and the native American Indians have used it for medicinal purposes for at least five hundred years. When I started prescribing it, almost twenty-five years ago in Scotland, it was thought to be an entirely new product and regarded with suspicion, until a medical research group began to show great interest in one of my patients, because she was recovering so quickly.

It is only recently that evening primrose oil has gained recognition as a valuable nutrient source. As I explained in Chapter Two, it is high in gammalinolenic acid (GLA), the precursor for prostaglandins which controls many biological functions. GLA production in humans can be affected by many factors, including saturated fats, sugars and alcohol. This explains why evening primrose oil is so important as a dietary supplement. I often ask teenagers suffering from acne vulgaris why they insist on eating sugar and chocolate, as the answer to their problems often lies in their diet. Certain foods must be considered off limits, and in the majority of cases it would help if the patient refrained from eating dairy products, nuts, chocolate, pork and related products, bananas, tomatoes, onions and citrus fruits. It may look a long list, but it will be worth their while to avoid these foods. In some persistent cases I may also ask if an acne patient is prepared to cut out wheat from the diet for a period of time. Wheat mostly aggravates an acne condition and many happy teenagers as well as adults, who were prepared to follow this advice, today no longer suffer from this problem.

Don't wash facial skin with soap and water. It is very much better to use a good quality skin cleanser, cleansing milk, or a mild soap. An excellent preparation from Nature's Best is the NaPCA Skin Moisturiser. Without NaPCA (Sodium Pyrrolidone Carboxylate) the skin would resemble dried and withered leaves. NaPCA is a natural moisturiser and humectant present in the skin. This means that it attracts moisture to the skin from the air, thus making it ideal for maintaining a soft and young-looking complexion. Nature's Best NaPCA is ideally suited for people of all ages, but since we lose up to 50 per cent of our natural NaPCA as we get older, it can be particularly useful in later years.

For a night cream I would suggest using vitamin E and Aloe Vera Cream, as Aloe Vera provides thorough skin care. This compound is extracted from the leaves of a desert cactus and contains vitamin C and many micro-nutrients. Each jar contains 5000 IU of vitamin E with 5ml of Aloe Vera Gel in a neutral base. For normal skin protection, I very often advise Annecy All-Purpose Cream as a day cream. This versatile moisturiser and sunscreen contains a sun protection factor of six and is suitable for indoor and outdoor use. PABA and NaPCA, two of nature's most beneficial skin care moisturisers, combined with Aloe Vera Gel, jojoba extract and Beta Carotene provide a really thorough all-purpose skin cream.

The structure and functions of the skin are of great importance to the overall health of the human body. A healthy skin often means a healthy body. The health of the skin is affected by a variety of factors – sunlight, dry air, extreme temperatures and chemical additives. It is therefore very important that we pay proper attention to the skin in order to keep it in as perfect a condition as possible, as a true reflection of our inner health.

Female patients in particular often enquire if their acne problem would be overcome more quickly or easily if they were to use hormonal products. Anything we do to encourage hormonal balance is important, but it should be done naturally. With all the science we have in this world, we still cannot claim to completely understand the hormonal system. With this in mind I would advise that, rather than using hormonal preparations which we really do not know enough about, it is always better to choose natural means, if that is at all possible.

The endocrine system is very important, especially with regard to acne. To help the endocrine system, in order to achieve the correct hormonal secretions and balance, it is essential to take evening primrose oil and certain vitamins. Walking, jogging and breathing exercises are also helpful. There are twenty or more little nerve centres situated in the solar plexus, with nerves extending to the different organs of the body, so deep breathing is relaxing as well as stimulating. Little veins accompany the nerves, carrying the blood to the different parts of the organs. Breathing exercises are good for minor hormonal disturbances, and, by consciously breathing deeply into the solar plexus, immediate contact is made with the different nerve centres, sending the nerve energy through to open up congestion, giving arteries a chance to force red blood and natural heat into the body and on to the various locations that may have been isolated. Try placing the left hand first on the solar plexus, then cover this hand with the right, and you form a magnetic ring. Breathe in and out slowly. For those of you who would like to develop this concept further, more detailed advice on breathing and other exercises can be found in my books *Stress and Nervous Disorders* and *Body Energy*. Such exercises are excellent as a general promoting influence for the nervous system.

As I mentioned earlier, the nervous system is made up of

two parts; the involuntary and sympathetic systems. The more you can relax this busy hormonal housekeeping, the more you relax the nerves, and the skin will flourish. A little time, effort and thought, will go a long way towards overcoming unwanted acne problems.

Now I turn to a very much bigger problem, which can be equally persistent, but much more difficult to control. This is *Acne rosacea*, a chronic disease of the skin affecting the fleshy areas of the face, the nose, cheeks, chin and forehead, occurring in both sexes, usually in middle life. This condition is caused by neurovascular instability, endocrine disorders, gastro-intestinal conditions, food problems, infections, alcoholism, allergies, and various other factors. I remember that Acne rosacea was once briefly mentioned in a Gloria Hunniford programme on BBC Radio 2. When we discussed this problem I had no idea of the hundreds of letters that would reach me from people looking for an answer to this particular problem. Although over the years I have seen quite a number of cases in my practice, I did not realise that there were so many sufferers, hence the reason that I decided to set aside a section for it in this chapter.

In recent times our eating habits have changed considerably and this is probably the reason behind the large number of Acne rosacea cases, and I have had many requests for help from people who had previously attended skin clinics and dermatologists and yet had not found a cure. I have achieved my most notable successes by concentrating on clearing the lymphatic system. In doing so I have discovered that severely inflamed cases cleared especially quickly. For all of us it would be wise to give some consideration to the lymphatic system, which performs a miraculous job, much of it during our sleeping hours. Considering its influence and importance, I will try to explain why the lymphatic system is under such threat.

Environmental and air pollution, the waste material from our food, and the toxic substances we often inhale, are all detrimental to the lymphatic system. To counteract these influences which can hardly be eliminated by the individual, Dr Vogel has developed an excellent remedy, Kelpasan, to assist the lymph glands to function properly. Kelpasan is made from pure sea algae from the Pacific Ocean and, as a food supplement, it stimulates the cell metabolism of the endocrine glands. It is also an excellent detoxifier and indeed, in its role as a detoxification method for the lymph system, it is of great help.

The lymphatics, which need ample rest and sleep, are more numerous than the arteries and veins, and are connected with all parts of the internal organs. They pass through the skin of the body, face and scalp, and also have a strong influence on the thyroid gland. They carry sensory action to all parts of the body; for example, the sense of taste – good or bad – is affected by the condition of the lymph. The lymph system is also decisive in the action or movement in any part of our neck or hands. If the lymph system becomes heavy and sluggish, it gradually slows the action of the blood, as it is the task of these glands to strengthen the red blood supply. The more active the lymph, the more quickly the body will move.

The lymphatic system consists of a complex network which collects the lymph from various organs and tissues in the human body. It is a system of inter-connecting vessels which conduct the lymph from the different parts of the body to the large veins of the neck, connecting with the jugular and other less important veins, where the lymph is poured into the bloodstream. In the system of connecting vessels there are many lymph glands or nodes. These small nodes or sacs, which act as filters and separate one substance from another, resemble buttons on a string, placed at different distances apart. Starting from the head and face, if we draw an imaginary line from the throat back to meet the third cervical vertebra, which is the bone in the middle of the neck, we find these strings of lymphatic nodes occurring closer to the surface of the skin on the face. One branch, occupying the skin, travels up the jaw to the eye, while two other branches travel to the nose. Two important nodes lie between the ear and the cheek bone in a line from the ear to the point of the nose. From here the glands, fifteen to twenty in number, travel up both sides of the head. The role of these glands is to collect fats and waste material and carry them into the deeper regions of the body. Just above the collar bone, on either side of the neck, we find a group of small nodes, five or six on either side, extending down into the deeper part of the body with branches extending down through the flesh and connecting with the shoulders. These little nodes can be felt in many parts of the body.

The next group is located in the back of the neck, travelling up inside the skull, forming a drainage system from the four different parts, and continuing from there down to the lower extremes of the body. Heat control in the body depends greatly on the action of these lymphatic nodes.

If we direct our attention to the lymphatic system in the neck, starting beneath the chin and travelling along the two main arteries down the breastbone or sternum, there is a group of lymphatics descending from the collar bone to the solar plexus. There is a little string of lymph nodes, or buttons, that seem to extend from the spinal column, sending out or collecting branches to and from the various parts of the flesh and diaphragm. Now, when we return to just below the collar bone, we find a large knob with branches running in different directions, travelling beneath the flesh and extending into the armpits. From there many lymphatic veins travel down the arms on both sides, but the largest group inhabit the palms of the hands and fingers. Here, by feeling, we notice the relation between the lymphatic group and the conscious system which carries every sense of vibration in the body.

The next group of lymphatics extends from the shoulders and is seated more deeply in the flesh, extending down the trunk of the body, with branches going to the breast. The entire breast area is one solid network of glands, with the exception of the nipples. This network of lymphatics is of great influence on the mammary glands. In the lower part of the back, in the lumbar region, we find a large lymphatic gland similar to an artery. At this point the gland branches out and has approximately twelve nodes. Other strings of nodes extend down into the lower part of the body to the fallopian tubes, ovarian glands, uterus, vagina, and lower limbs. These glands collect the lymph from the lower extremities and carry it in the direction of the heart. There it connects with one of the main arteries and pours the lymph and chyle milk, which is a milky substance, into the blood. The lymph is carried around by the circulation of the red blood until the blood passes through the kidneys, where the detrimental substances are extracted and eliminated by the force of the urine channels.

Because so many problems can be traced back to the lymphatic system, I have tried to explain it in detail. It is the lymphatic system that is responsible for the proper elimination of waste material, and, accordingly, its functions affect the condition of skin and flesh of the body. It has been established that the lymphatic system will not flourish without adequate calcium supplies, and in many acne rosacea patients I have discovered a chronic calcium deficiency. The calcium preparation I mostly prescribe is called Urticalcin from the Bioforce range, as I believe that this is one of the most easily absorbed calcium supplements. Not only is this a homoeopathic supplement, so that there is no need to fear calcium deposits, but it is also mixed with nettle extract – *Herb urtica*. Urticalcin, as a homoeopathic calcium and silicic acid preparation, is to be used where a deficiency is indicated.

Another very important factor is dietary management. The tongue is entirely covered with a network of lymphatic veins or glands, large groups occupying the centre of the tongue. As the lymphatic system is closely linked with the conscious system, which is a system of cell tissue encasing the flesh throughout the entire body, the lymphatic system is dependent upon a healthy diet. In cases of acne rosacea

59

all very hot foods or drinks, especially caffeine-containing drinks, should be forbidden. Alcohol and food allergens such as coffee, chocolate, tea, milk and pork can aggravate the problem. I also want to see citrus fruits mentioned in the list of prohibited food, as I have noticed that the condition usually deteriorates as a result of eating oranges, lemons or grapefruit. An acne rosacea sufferer should also be careful of intense sunshine, and would be wise to seek the shade. Extra vitamins should be taken and I would advise large quantities of vitamin C, at least one or two grammes per day.

Individual requirements and levels of vitamin C vary, dependent upon external and environmental factors, personal circumstances and each individual's biochemical make-up. Unusually busy periods in life can increase the requirement for this vitamin. Many smokers, those taking aspirins, antibiotics and the contraceptive pills, and alcohol drinkers, ought to consider supplementing vitamin C. Menstruating women and the elderly often require extra vitamin C, and during pregnancy and lactation the need for vitamin C is increased.

Man cannot manufacture ascorbic acid (vitamin C), which is so important for body chemistry, within the body and therefore it is important to ensure that the supply is adequate. Its main functions include:
– The maintenance of collagen which is a glue-like protein that connects our skin, ligaments and tissues.
– It is a powerful anti-oxidant, preventing damage to tissues, membranes and cells.
– Regulation of cholesterol levels in the body.
– Protection of the immune system.

Vitamin C is the least stable of the vitamins as it is water soluble and easily lost from the body. This makes it necessary to ensure that we get an adequate supply on a daily basis. To maintain a high level of vitamin C in the bloodstream at all times, small frequent intakes are better than one single large dose, because excess vitamin C is excreted from the body within three hours of ingestion.

I would also advise taking potassium, as this distributes intra-cellular fluids. Sodium is found in the highest incidence of extra cellular fluids. The distribution of both minerals helps to maintain the fluid balance of the body. Potassium is also essential for protein and carbohydrate metabolism, which, for this condition, is essential. At all times oil of evening primrose and vitamins A and D can be taken as these will help to overcome acne conditions more quickly.

At night I would advise applying some Bioforce Seven Herb Cream on the affected areas. This is a healing cream containing seven different herbal extracts, combined with avocado oil, lanolin and other oils, plus beeswax. Due to this lubricating base, Bioforce Seven Herbs Cream soothes, softens and nourishes the skin, while promoting its health. As a day cream I would recommend Echinacea cream, which I have already mentioned because of its antiseptic and antibiotic properties.

For the scalp I recommend that a teaspoonful of Molkosan is added to the final rinsing water when shampooing the hair, as this helps to calm the itchiness, while also clearing the scalp.

In summary, my advice to acne rosacea patients would be to use Echinaforce, Petasan, and occasionally some of the creams or supplements mentioned above. Remember that with this particular skin condition, natural treatment very often supplies an answer where orthodox treatment may have failed. Don't despair if no immediate improvement is obvious. Never give up hope and persevere with the treatment.

5

Skin Infections

THE LIST of possible skin infections seems endless and some are more serious than others. Yet, they all require attention and in order to decide on the correct treatment it is important to find out what type of infection we are dealing with and, better still, how this infection may have originated. It is possible that it is *Impetigo* or a *Cutaneous tuberculosis*. Whatever, never neglect even a minor scratch that refuses to heal, or a sore that does not reduce in size: the body tells us in its own way that it needs attention. Bear in mind that the skin is formed from the same layer *in utero* as the nervous system, and is indeed an extension of the nervous system.

In an earlier chapter I pointed out the possible relationship between skin infections and the lymphatic system. Nowadays the lymphatic system is often overloaded with waste material, with which it very often cannot cope. The health and condition of the skin will always be vastly improved by improving the flow of the lymphatic system and to this end, simple methods, such as brushing or gently massaging the skin towards the heart, drinking red clover tea, hydrotherapy techniques as in different forms of bathing, the use of Epsom salts to draw out the superficial toxins, or a handful of bicarbonate of soda in the bathwater, are often beneficial. Remember though, always take a shower after having bathed in these salts. Finish with a hot shower, ending with a spray of cold water on the lower limbs. In my book *Water – Healer or Poison?*, much other useful information can be found to help cases of skin problems. This book contains quite a number of treatments according to the methods advocated by Father Kneipp, such as chamomile and hay baths, which are all excellent methods to improve one's skin condition.

A further important factor in all skin conditions, and this is a relatively modern influence, is stress. I often relate to my patients 'the three S's', which are obstacles to good health: salt, sugar and stress. The emotional background of stress in particular, is likely to aggravate any dormant skin condition. The stress factor should never be ignored. In the first place, stress depletes our potassium supplies, essential to everyone's health, and it eats away at our reserves of various vitamins, minerals and trace elements. Especially in the case of skin conditions caused by allergies, the influence of stress becomes very clear. I have written about this in more detail in my book *Viruses, Allergies and the Immune System*, where I have emphasised the fact that stress influences the texture of one's skin. I take this opportunity to repeat that the skin is an external indicator of the internal condition of the body.

When very severe skin conditions are experienced, e.g. *Scleroderma*, where the entire surface of the skin is being threatened by hardening or calcifying, it is my experience that this condition can be improved by reducing the stress factor. Under such, or similar, conditions the patient would be wise to consider relaxation methods. Relaxation can be achieved in a variety of ways, such as breathing exercises, water exercises, or muscular relaxation exercises, which are all acceptable suggestions for improving infectious conditions.

Under such circumstances detoxification is also important and this can be achieved by various fasting programmes. For such conditions Dr Vogel's remedy Echinaforce is most helpful: take 15 drops in a little water three times a day. It also makes sense to take some Bioflavonoids, as these remedies are applicable for all inflammatory conditions. Supplements of vitamins A, C and E, and the minerals zinc, chromium and selenium are also beneficial. Dr Vogel has great faith in the use of clay for many forms of skin infection, and this can be used effectively in a number of different ways. In recent years I more frequently advise the use of Beta Carotene, as I have found that this will improve any skin conditions and skin infections in particular. I am a great believer in looking at the improvements resulting from the use of certain remedies, as such knowledge may be helpful in other cases. In certain cases the acceptable treatment may not be successful and then I may decide to prescribe a different combination of treatments which appeared to have been applicable to a closely related condition.

Grey and pasty skin indicates problems with the liver, gallbladder and lymphatic system. *Acne vulgaris* or *Acne rosacea* indicates liver or pancreas problems, or possibly that the bowel needs some special attention. A blotchy skin may suggest a congested liver. Skin that reminds us of crepe paper often indicates a deficiency of fatty acids. Thinning of the skin, especially after the menopause, shows a poor adrenal oestrogen production. Skin reminiscent of fish scales may be the result of one of many causes, but it is always in desperate need of essential fatty acids. For cracked feet problems, although incurable, the function of the gallbladder and the liver should receive special attention. Athlete's foot is very often diagnosed as a *Candida syndrome*. Scalp problems such as dandruff, cradle cap, and general thinning of the hair, usually indicate a defective protein absorption and a chronic lack of minerals, and this diagnosis is also applicable when the finger- and toenails break easily or split into different layers, so weakening the nails. Small bumps on the back of the arms appear as the result of a vitamin A deficiency, caused by the liver not functioning correctly. A very dry and lumpy skin may be caused by a water deficiency, while sore skin may result from lymph congestion. All these symptoms are an indication that something, somewhere, is not as it should be.

Now let's turn to some specific skin infections. Lately I have noticed a gradual increase in *Impetigo*. The lesions of this contagious skin infection are characterised by thin, rolled vesicles or pustules, in a thick superficial crust, often caused by haemolytic streptococcus and staphylococcus influences. To my mind *impetigo* is caused more often nowadays by a faulty diet than by poor hygienic management. In hot climates *impetigo* problems seem to be becoming more common and there I think the causes lie in diet and hygiene in equal importance. Fortunately, *impetigo* can be cleared relatively easily, as long as the right measures are taken.

With children in particular, one should look at the child's constitutional condition and likely causes will be malnutrition or a poorly balanced diet. Introduce plenty of fruit and vegetables into the diet and consider substituting cow's milk with goat's milk. Try to make the child eat raw food, such as salads, although I admit that this may not be so easy in younger cildren. Added to this, bathing in Epsom Salts baths and the use of Echinaforce, Violaforce and Urticalcin, makes a very good all-round treatment to clear *impetigo*.

A similar treatment programme can be used for *Erysipelas*, which is an acute infection of the skin caused by a haemolytic streptococcus, usually displaying red swollen areas with some 'flu-like symptoms and inflammation. The streptococcus bacteria lies at the root of many problems and infections caused by this bacteria should not be underestimated:

treatment should be undertaken immediately on discovery. The American doctor Edward Rosenow has specialised his research in viral infections for over sixty years. Since 1925 he has written and published more than 450 medical papers, mainly on the subject of the effects of different viruses on the body. Dr Rosenow has discussed the streptococcus bacteria on several occasions and believes that millions of organisms exist in the human body, although a specific streptococcus bacteria is responsible for many diseases. He also discovered the strength of streptococcus, stating that to destroy this bacteria, it took 19 hours of boiling in H_2O_2 (hydrogen peroxide). Such is its strength that it can maintain life in temperatures ranging from 350 degrees Fahrenheit to minus 150 degrees Fahrenheit. He also found that it is so small that a trillion of this virus can live in one square centimetre alongside other bacteria. Both of these facts show what formidable opposition we are up against.

Although an Erysipelas condition can be cured relatively quickly, one must never underestimate the strength and influence of a streptococcus infection in any skin disease. Its characteristics are shining skin lesions which can cause much damage and, although the area of inflammation may be small, it can be very persistent. Always make sure that exact hygiene measures are maintained and, wherever possible, disposable materials should be used and immediately disposed off and destroyed. A high dose of vitamins is recommended, especially vitamin A together with Health Insurance Plus, Echinaforce and Petasan. It is also important to ensure a good flow of urine. Drink ample amounts of fluid and make sure that there is no restriction or blockage of the urine flow and, to this end, a natural diuretic may be advisable. A good natural diuretic, for example, is asparagus and celery used with some Solidago (Golden Rod) as a herbal remedy.

Yet another persistent problem that is occurring more frequently, is *Herpes simplex*, sometimes referred to as fever blister, cold sore, or *Herpes menstrualis*. This acute virus infection can be a downright nuisance, and a frequently recurring plague. An individual or multiple infection, filled with clear fluid and raised in an inflammatory base, occurs on the skin, the mucous membranes and the conjunctiva. This infection can easily occur in infancy or among young people and the local areas of infection can be very irritable, depending how often they occur and the manifestation of the variety. Usually the mouth and lips are affected, but inflammation can also appear on the extremities. Some severe reactions can take place and treatment becomes more difficult when it affects the eyes, the cornea, the nose, cheeks, elbows, or even the vagina, which sometimes causes extreme and persistent discomfort. *Genital herpes* is also an ever-increasing and very persistent problem. I recognise that this is most uncomfortable, but it can be cured.

An even more difficult condition for the sufferer is *Kaposi syndrome*, as its eruptions can lead to many problems. Although it is often said that there is no cure for this condition, I disagree. Over the years I have found that with Herpes simplex and even Kaposi syndrome, herbal treatments and the use of vitamins, minerals and trace elements are extremely helpful. The best supplement for such conditions, to my mind, is Multiple Four Plus. This is a unique supplement containing more than fifty different ingredients, including vitamins, minerals, amino acids, herbs, sea vegetables and enzymes. The formula includes digestive aids to promote efficient uptake of nutrients from food, making Multiple Four Plus an unusually supportive supplement. The tablets are hypo-allergenic and free from wheat, yeast, gluten, and artificial colours, flavourings and preservatives. It is advisable to take one or two tablets with meals, depending on the circumstances and requirements.

Each tablet provides the following impressive list:

Vitamin A Palmitate	5,500 IU	Copper (as Gluconate)	0.5 mg
Vitamin D₃	225 IU	Iron (as Fumarate)	5 mg
Vitamin C (Calcium Ascorb)	125 mg	Magnesium (as Gluconate)	56 mg
Vitamin B₁ (Thiamin)	7 mg	Manganese (as Gluconate)	13 mg
Vitamin B₂ (riboflavin)	7 mg	Potassium (as Gluconate)	15 mg
Vitamin B₆ (Pyridoxine HCl)	9 mg	Selenium (as Seleno-Methionine)	8 mcg
Vitamin B₁₂	15 mcg	Zinc (as Gluconate)	8 mg
Vitamin E d-Alpha	55 IU	Bladderwrack	17 mg
Biotin	38 mcg	Cascara Sagrada	17 mg
Calcium Pantothenate	38 mg	Cayenne	17 mg
Choline (as Bitartrate)	50 mg	Comfrey	19 mg
Bioflavonoids	25 mg	Dandelion Root	17 mg
Folic Acid	100 mcg	Golden Seal	17 mg
Nicotinic Acid	15 mg	Horsetail Grass	17 mg
Nicotinamide	30 mg	Saw Palmetto Berries	17 mg
Inositol	25 mg	Iron Ox Bile	8 mg
PABA	8 mg	Pancrelipase	8 mg
Rutin	7 mg	RNA	15 mg
Hesperidin Complex	14 mg	Bromelain	7 mg
Iodine (as Potassium Iodide)	67 mcg	Betain HCl	7 mg
L-Methionine	1 mg	Papain	7 mg
Almond Powder	18 mg	Liver concentrate	26 mg
Calcium (as Gluconate)	10 mg	Yellow Dock	17 mg
Chromium (as Orotate)	13 mcg	Lecithin	38 mg

It is also worthwhile drinking herbal teas, such as Chamomile, Golden Seal, Saxifrage, or a mixture that combines all of them: the Jan de Vries 100 per cent Herbal Health Tea. With regard to diet, it would be wise to adopt a cleansing diet regime and take some extra Acidopholus or drink buttermilk. Do not eat fried or deep-fried food, sugar in any form, white bread, dry cereal, canned food, coffee, or alcohol. To do this for even a short time will help greatly towards controlling a herpes condition.

Genital warts can also be very persistent and the only way to rid oneself of these undesirable and unpleasant skin eruptions is to use the dietary management described above, and take Petasan and Chelidonium. The latter is a fresh herb preparation for the cauterisation of warts and wart-like growths. It can be used internally, three times a day, ten drops in a little water, but it is also very helpful to dab some of this fluid with a piece of cottonwool on the affected area. The worst case of genital warts I have been asked to treat took almost twelve months to clear. It can be a very difficult and persistent condition, but one should never give up hope. Apart from dabbing with Chelidonium, one can also use Molkosan. In its pure extract form this is very helpful for genital warts, although occasionally it may be too strong, in which case it may have to be diluted slightly.

This brings me to the problem of *warts*. These must be treated quickly to prevent the onset of a fast-spreading and possibly prolonged condition. Thuja is an excellent homoeopathic remedy for internal use, and if this does not resolve the situation, there are various other herbal remedies that can be used. Warts can be readily transmitted between people and can appear on any part of the body. They sometimes disappear voluntarily, but to prevent spreading, immediate action should be taken. Other homoeopathic preparations that may be used under such circumstances are Calcium Carbonica or Sepia, but dabbing with Chelidonium will always be helpful. Castor oil can also be used for gentle dabbing on the affected areas and occasionally I have found this to be a useful alternative in the treatment of warts, as well as in the even more persistent, wart-like condition, *veruccae*.

A *verruca* is a type of wart, caused by a virus infection of the skin. It may occur anywhere on the body, but is usually found on the feet or hands. *Verrucae* are extremely contagious and you may become infected by going barefoot where someone else with a *verruca* has walked. This could be a swimming pool, a changing room, or a gymnasium. It may take several months for the infection to show. A virus is far too small to be seen with the naked eye, but you will certainly not miss the effects of the *verruca* virus on the skin. If one is lucky it may be contained to a single verruca, yet it is equally possible that there will be a patch of them.

Because the virus infects the cells of the skin, whichever treatment is selected, some skin cells may require to be destroyed in the process and this may cause some discomfort for a period of time. No two infections are the same and the most effective treatment to suit you will be selected by your chiropodist. Occasionally he may even decide that the verruca does not require treatment. Trust his judgement. If your chiropodist decides that treatment is required, he can decide on any of the following methods:

Cryosurgery

This involves holding a very cold probe against the *verruca* for a time varying from one to three minutes which may be in two spells. You may be given a local anaesthetic injection near the *verruca*. If not, the freezing will hurt somewhat. Expect the verruca to throb for two or three hours after the treatment. You may even develop a blister or a blood blister within the first week. If this is uncomfortable, let your chiropodist know and he will deal with this. Otherwise you need take no precautions and your feet are allowed to get wet. It is customary that your chiropodist asks you back for a check-up after approximately four weeks.

Electrosurgery

This method involves burning or cutting away the verruca, using electrical power. With this treatment method you should always be given a local anaesthetic in the area near the verruca.

Excision

This treatment consists of cutting away the affected skin, also after having received a local anaesthetic.

When the injection wears off, the site may be a little tender and there may be some bleeding. You will be asked to keep the foot dry for two or three days, or until the bleeding has stopped. Keep the verruca covered for this time. If there is a lot of bleeding, you must let the chiropodist know. Under normal circumstances he will ask you to see him again in one week's time for a check-up.

If you prefer non-surgical treatment for a verruca, dab the area with castor oil or Chelidonium. Again, Thuja may be taken. Allow me to point out once again that natural cures have much to offer and, as always, a good cleansing diet is important.

6

Fungal Conditions

IT CAN be very embarrassing when you have to shake someone's hand when that hand shows a fungal condition. This usually displays itself in the palm of the hand, where the skin feels hard and is of a reddish, cracked texture. Fungal conditions can be persistent and difficult to treat. They often start on the hands, or sometimes on the feet, as in the case of *athlete's foot*, or on some remote areas of the skin. They can be recognised by skin eruptions, inflammation, and cracked skin.

Not so long ago I had a patient with a fungal condition on the hands, and whatever I recommended, no progress was made. I mentioned this case to my old teacher, Dr Alfred Vogel. He told me that at one time he had visited the Javaras, an Indian tribe, where he had noticed many incidences of skin fungi, and went on to tell me how they treated their people: there, in the wild, originated today's remedy, Spilanthes.

Spilanthes Oleracea or *Paracress* is a fresh herbal preparation to be used externally in cases of fungal conditions and infections. For a fungus within the mouth, this is also a wonderful remedy. In such instances, Spilanthes can be used as a mouth rinse for the inflammation of the mucous membranes, when it is recommended that at least 40 or 50 drops are used. For skin fungal conditions, including those under the finger- and toenails, it is advisable to dab *Spilanthes* on the affected areas two or three times a day.

Usually when I treat a patient for a fungus, I recommend the use of Petasan and Molkosan, both remedies from the Bioforce range. Molkosan is produced from fresh Alp whey, by a natural fermentation process. It contains all the important minerals found in fresh whey, such as magnesium, potassium and calcium in a concentrated form. Molkosan is also rich in natural dextrorotatory lactic acid, which in health-oriented nutrition, as well as natural healing methods, has a specific significance. Molkosan can also be used in the preparation of salad dressings, but for therapeutic purposes I recommend that twice a day, half a teaspoonful is drunk diluted in half a glass of water. This is beneficial for a healthy intestinal flora, and for any external skin condition, even for minor cuts and abrasions, but also for a persistent condition like athlete's foot. This condition can be very difficult to treat, but even here Molkosan has proved helpful.

Athlete's foot is probably the most commonly known fungus disease and can be very widespread. The skin frequently becomes raw and eroded, with a burning and itching feeling, and, as a result of touching, it can affect the hands too. Readers who have first-hand experience of this skin disease are bound to agree that it is a difficult condition to treat. However, Spilanthes and Molkosan for external treatment, and Petasan for internal use, will be of great help.

Ringworm, or *Tinea Favosa*, also called 'honeycomb' or *Porrigo Scutula*, affects mainly the scalp, the nails, and a few other parts of the skin. It generally starts with some scaling and crusting and is likely to leave some scar damage. This condition also requires immediate attention and, again, I mostly recommend the use of Echinaforce and Urticalcin, as these remedies will help to get the condition quickly under control. If the scaly patches are itchy, dab the areas with Molkosan. This is also helpful for *barber's itch* (or ringworm of the beard). Sometimes this condition starts very gradually, but once it has had a chance to establish itself, the inflammatory process can spread rapidly over the area covered by a beard. It can be a source of great embarrassment when the hairs become dry and brittle, break off, and nasty scaly patches become visible.

With any of the aforementioned conditions it makes good sense to provide some extra help for the immune system. Immunity is very important at the best of times, as an effective immune system provides the most effective defence against any foreign agents, which may attack the body in a variety of ways. Although the immune system is complex and capable of exerting multiple effects, the condition of the immune system does depend largely on how well it is looked after. Despite ample research into this aspect of our health, many questions still remain unanswered. Nevertheless, it is safe to say that the best way to build up and strengthen the immune system is the natural way. A balanced natural diet and the use of supplementary vitamins, minerals and trace elements will always help us to better withstand infections, fungi, viruses or parasites. If we could be sure that our diet was well balanced, we would not need to take supplements. However, doctors and nutritionists are in agreement that it is rare that all the basic requirements are provided in our diet.

In an excellent article in *The Times* of 6 April 1992, I read that the US Government has adopted 1990 dietary guidelines, urging an ambitious, varied meal plan: three to five servings daily of vegetables, two to four of fruit, as well as six to eleven containing bread, rice, pasta or grains. Despite all this dietary help, people still need supplementary vitamins, minerals and trace elements, largely because, due to modern agricultural methods, our food may not meet the nutritional requirements our modern lifestyle demands of the body. Fortunately the same article continued to state that, thanks to new research, ever more scientists now believe that traditional medical views on vitamins and minerals have been too limited. While researchers may not endorse the expansive claims of the hard-core vitamin enthusiasts, evidence suggests that nutrients play a much more complex role in assuring vitality and optimum health than was previously thought. Vitamins, often in doses much higher than those usually recommended, may protect us from a host of ills, ranging from birth defects and cataracts, to heart disease and cancer. Even more provocative are glimmerings that vitamins can stave off the normal ravages of ageing. It is revealing that this article put the emphasis on the use of vitamins. Certainly, to help the immune system, a healthy well-balanced diet is necessary, as well as, in many cases, the use of extra vitamins.

The same article also stated that food contains a myriad of obscure nutrients, such as phenols, flafones and luteins. This is something scientists cannot yet fully understand, much less put into a safe and effective pill form, and undoubtedly many more nutrients have not even been identified yet. Even if a full-service nutrient pill were formulated, it would probably not be able to satisfy some basic home desires, like hunger and the joy of savouring food. It is quite heartening to think that the time has arrived when we are ready to admit that an inadequate food pattern may demonstrate itself in skin disorders, indicating that internally something is deficient.

In the past, when the word immunity was used, it usually referred to the phenomena wherein, having been infected with a disease, it was unlikely that the same condition would recur. However, in recent years social problems, caused by specific infections, have become the topic of widespread discussion and speculation. Since then, immunity in general has become associated with the body's defence mechanism, and not only for infectious diseases. As a result the importance attached to immunity has allowed a widening of the prophylaxis of therapy for many disorders. How an organism is maintained in a certain state depends on various mechanisms for its protection. Even external enemies will threaten life in an immunological mechanism. Immunological cells may be reduced both quantatively and qualitatively due to many factors, and we live in times when the immunological ability must be constantly reinforced. In this matter we can have considerable influence, if we are so inclined.

We can start by accepting the need and responsibility for a balanced and nutritional diet. We can decide to follow a sensible exercising programme. We can also judge if the level of stress we personally experience is acceptable or not. If the latter is the case, we can seek advice on how to deal with, or reduce it. Rest assured that by taking positive action the immune system will be reinforced. Moreover, preparations are available that have been devised for the specific purpose of strengthening the immune system, such as Imunoforce from the Bioforce range and Imuno-Strength, which I have formulated myself for Nature's Best. Imuno-Strength is able to deal with viruses, bacteria and toxins, before they become established. Today's world is full of challenges to our defence mechanisms. Some of these are under our control – such as the food we eat, the stresses and strains of work – others are not. These include environmental pollution by potentially toxic chemicals. In these circumstances it makes sense to help protect the integrity of our immune system by safeguarding our nutrition. Nature's Best has been able to go one better with a special formula. As well as carefully selected amounts of vitamins and minerals known to be needed for proper functioning of the immune system, Imuno-Strength contains the herbs Devil's Claw and Echinacea.

Each tablet contains:

Vitamin A	900 mcg	Iron	1 mg
	(3000 IU)	Magnesium	3 mg
Riboflavin (vitamin B_2)	10 mg	Manganese	500 mcg
Vitamin B_6	50 mg	Selenium	100 mcg
Folic Acid	50 mcg	Zinc	20 mg
Pantothenic Acid	50 mg	Devil's Claw	100 mg
Vitamin C	165 mg	Echinacea Purpurea	200 mg
Vitamin E	80 IU	Thymus Concentrate	15 mg
Calcium	19 mg	Siberian Ginseng	15 mg

The golden rule is to consider the importance of the immune system, not only in the case of fungal conditions, but for other skin disorders as well. If in any doubt as to whether your immune system may need help, don't delay. Do something about it as soon as possible.

7

Abscesses

AN *ABSCESS* can be an extremely uncomfortable and painful affliction. An abscess is often an accumulation of internal and external material and a sure sign that the patient has a high level of toxicity. Usually the lymphatic system collects and disposes of most of the waste material, but sometimes it may not be able to cope with excessive demands. When this happens some of this waste material may seek its own way of escape. Unfortunately, quite often any excess is the result of an unbalanced or unsuitable diet, although it can also be due to specific poisonous material, or smoking or drinking too much. This invasive material is gathered in the lymph glands and if these glands cannot cope with its disposal or discharge, it will accumulate into an abscess that may appear at random anywhere on the surface of the body.

If an abscess is a recurring chronic condition, everything must be done to eliminate the toxic waste from the body. Lancing or operating on the abscess will bring relief, but the cause will not be removed, and there should be an investigation into why toxicity stretches the lymphatic system beyond its limits. External treatment does not eliminate the underlying toxins and it is only by treating the cause of the problem that the patient can be certain this will not be a regular recurrence.

A patient who once came to see me, admitted that she had reached the point of despair as she continuously suffered from abscesses under the arms. She had even consented to have some of her lymph glands removed in the hope that this would stop the formation of abscesses, but it was all to no avail. External abscesses are hard to deal with, but it is even more difficult to correctly diagnose internal abscesses, and these can occur on any of the vital organs, such as the lungs or the liver. Again, this is certain proof of a highly toxic system.

I apologise if I appear to be repeating myself, but it is possible to rid the body of such toxins, if only we start with the basics, namely good dietary management. The lady in question had all along refused to accept this fact and determinedly continued to smoke. Her diet also contained far too much sugar and in the end, when even the surgical operation proved non-effective, she was sufficiently desperate to find a cure that she eventually agreed to reduce her smoking and consider a change in her diet.

She cut back her smoking drastically and agreed to certain dietary changes that I suggested, some of them being to avoid spices and junk food. Moreover, to improve her bowel movements, which used to cause her considerable problems, I suggested some colonic irrigation. Her lymph glands were swollen and the lymphatic system needed urgent attention. I am pleased to say that eventually I was visited by a very grateful patient, who looked years younger than when I first met her, and to her delight she had not had another abscess since. I told her that she had achieved this herself.

Boils or *carbuncles* are swellings of the skin, which often develop around the hair follicles. Sometimes there is just one, but often there are more. It is a painful condition and arising from toxins in the bloodstream, again mostly due to the wrong foods. In these cases the best course is often a revision of the diet, and frequently I also advise a period of fasting, as this allows the body to detoxify itself. I can assure you that any patient who suffers from boils or carbuncles with regularity, will be more than willing to co-operate. As always, proper elimination is necessary for good health. When the nervous system is confused by a misunderstanding of our physical ailments and our anatomy, the circulation of the blood is always interfered with and this, in turn, causes constipation. The framework of the body must be seen in its entirety and it is not only the bowels, the lymph glands, the nerves, the arteries or the veins that need help. It is possible, and even likely, that there are more than one or two factors that require attention.

This is also the case with *varicose veins* which result from blockage of the ventricles (or veins) that return the blood to the kidneys and heart. A circulatory system with abscesses, varicose veins or haemorrhoids, is usually a sign of an inefficient bowel function and diminished elimination. Some people tell me in all sincerity that they have no bowel problems, yet, when quizzed, they tell me that they have a bowel movement every second or third day. Nevertheless they don't consider this unusual. One of the basic rules of good health is that whatever is imported, ought to be exported within a period of twenty-four hours. Abscesses, boils, carbuncles, etc. cannot be expected to disappear unless the toxicity problem has been resolved.

An effective method to quickly remove the toxins from the body is a period of fasting on a grape diet, which means what it says, i.e. no other food than grapes should pass the lips. This diet should not be followed for longer than four days. An even more foolproof way to rid the body of toxins is by colonic irrigation. As more and more people begin to feel the benefits of colonic irrigation, it is becoming better known and more widely accepted as a therapeutic procedure. Yet, many people still know relatively little about this treatment method, so I will explain how and why the treatment is given, and what should or should not be done in colonic irrigation. A good friend of mine runs a clinic in Toronto, Canada, which specialises in colonic irrigation treatments, called Resto-Clean. Most of the following information is based on the procedures followed in that clinic.

Colonic irrigation is a means of restoring the colon to a healthy state so that it can perform its function properly. It involves a hygienic cleansing of the lower bowel, or large intestine, using water. The modern diet, on the whole, is too full of refined foods, saturated oils and chemical substances, which puts a strain on the whole body. Besides this, the stress of modern living and the environment in which we live, are conducive to creating disorders which place a great burden on the whole elimination system. This creates abnormal conditions which prevent the colon from working properly. A colon irrigation is done to clean it and restore it to its proper function.

The colon's main functions are to continue digestion of food started in the small intestine, to remove water for use by the body, and to convey waste and toxic material outside the body. It does the latter by means of waves of muscle contraction in the wall of the colon, called peristalsis. It also holds bacteria which begins the process of breaking down the waste into its components, thus preventing a toxic condition in the body. It should take no more than twenty-four hours for food to move through the digestive system. However, the colon handles more than the food we eat; it also expels the dead cells from the body. In other words, the colon is the body's sewage system.

Two common symptoms of colon trouble are constipation and diarrhoea. But there are many conditions which an unhealthy colon will produce, which appear to be unrelated to the colon. Since the colon is the whole body's sewage system, any problems which cause it to malfunction will have effects elsewhere. If waste builds up through constipation, a general condition which affects the whole body, called *toxaemia*, can occur, in which poisons from the colon are circulated through the bloodstream, giving rise to serious problems in several organs. Generally speaking though, problems in the colon show up in the digestive system first. Colon irrigation will help any condition which is caused by a back-up of poisons in the body. Since every organ throws off waste material, usually through the blood, an inability to dispose of the waste will poison the entire body.

As to the question of who should have colonic irrigation, it would be too easy to say 'Everyone'. Certainly anyone who has chronic problems in the digestive and/or elimination system should begin a series of treatments. They are not normally needed for small children, but treatment can be given to children over six years of age. The average person in our society, including children, has a diet which creates problems in the colon, whether or not he or she is aware of it. Even in a 'healthy' person, the walls of the colon become impacted with waste matter which builds up over a number of years. This prevents the efficient functioning of the colon. Any person with this condition will benefit from this treatment therapy.

A person with a colon which functions normally, should have about as many bowel movements per day as he or she had meals the previous day. There should be no constipation or diarrhoea. These things would seem to indicate a healthy colon. However, because the body organs are designed to function normally under some level of stress, the appearance of a healthy colon may mask a growing problem in the digestive system. Therefore, it is a good preventive measure to remove poisons and wastes and maintain good health by means of a cleansing of the lower bowel.

Ideally, colonics should be done by trained colon therapists, who have a good knowledge of the anatomy and physiology of the digestive system. A trained nurse is best. People who are untrained in colon therapy should be avoided.

There are different ways of performing colon irrigation. In this age of machinery one would expect that there is a machine to do the work, and indeed there is. But machines, even sophisticated ones, are not very sensitive to the human condition. These machines pump water into the bowel and let it drain several times. This is called a pressure method since the machine relies on an increase of pressure in the bowel to make it drain the water. A better method involves using gravity, rather than pressure. Gravity and the continuous and active involvement of a trained colon specialist makes this a gentler and far superior method of irrigation. In the gravity method, a tank of water located at a certain height above the patient (12–18 inches) provides adequate pressure through gravity and the manual control of the water allows a more individual treatment.

Colonics are done in a room housing a padded table for the patient to lie on, the colonic irrigation apparatus and a chair for the therapist. The therapist talks to new patients to explain the procedure and notes down a short medical history. Anyone who has not been referred by a physician, chiropractor or naturopath, will be asked to contact their doctor to determine whether there is any reason why colonic irrigation should not take place. If desired, the therapist may approach the doctor on behalf of the patient.

Patients are asked to empty the bladder prior to the treatment, because the bowel will be massaged. Setting up the equipment involves filling a five-gallon tank with water, taking the proctoscope from the steriliser, attaching the tubes to the proctoscope and lubricating it. Clients are asked to lie on their sides for the initial part of the irrigation and then on their backs. The water is set to a certain temperature, usually between 80 and 96 degrees Fahrenheit or 27 to 35 degrees Celsius, depending upon the condition of the bowel, and allowed to flow into the colon through a quarter-inch tube. By blocking the large exit tube, the therapist prevents water from flowing out and puts a little water into the colon. By releasing the exit tube, they allow the water to drain, carrying with it toxins, fecal matter, mucus, and fermentation and other debris from the colon. This is carried directly into the sewage system. By filling up the colon more and more on successive cycles, the whole colon is eventually cleaned. The therapist massages the colon upon releasing the water in order to encourage the expulsion of toxic waste. Often the colon will help in this by producing waves of muscle contractions, which is quite normal. The site of many toxins is the caecum at the end of the colon closest to the small intestine. One of the goals of the treatment is to irrigate this portion well and rid it of toxic waste. This is not always possible at first, depending upon the condition of, and blockage in, the bowel, but after a number of irrigation treatments all parts of the bowel are cleaned.

After going through this, 'fill, release, massage, empty' procedure several times and using about fifteen gallons of water, the treatment will be finished. It will have taken from half-an-hour to an hour. At the end of the treatment the proctoscope is removed and the client goes to the toilet to discharge any water left in the colon.

After colonic irrigation the patient should take acidophilus (yoghurt culture) capsules or tablets in order to ensure that the intestinal flora in the colon are replaced. If the patient has been referred by a chiropractor, naturopath or physician, the colon therapist's report to him, or her, may lead to a prescription for further herbal or drug treatments.

If we have a normally healthy colon, a series of twelve to sixteen irrigation treatments should be enough to bring it to a high level of efficiency. In the case of toxic colons, a longer series of treatment may be required.

A good diet and effort to eliminate or control stress and fatigue will keep us generally healthy, and good health means a well-functioning colon. Under these conditions colonic irrigation every three to six months will ensure that the body as a whole is kept clean and vital.

At the Toronto clinic an excellent system has been worked out and, on departure from the clinic, the patient is given post-treatment dietary recommendations to ensure optimum benefit from the colonic treatment. These recommendations are as follows:

Don't Eat
Red meats
Fried foods or oils
Salads and raw vegetables

Eat
All fruit (papaya, mango and pineapple are best for enzymes)
Cooked grains
Steamed vegetables
Soups
Juices
Sprouts
Chicken or fish (unless vegetarian)
N.B. After twenty-four hours raw vegetables and uncooked oils may be taken.

To promote elimination and digestion
Carrot, spinach, beet, or watermelon juices

Toxin-absorbing foods
Beets, watermelon, apples (or apple sauce), red grape juice

Vitamins E and C should also be used for colonic conditions. Vitamin E acts as an anti-oxidant and Nature's Best has selected the most potent and biologically active form of natural vitamin E to use in their supplements. Vitamin E (alpha tocopherol) is the most powerful vitamin in the body's anti-oxidant defence system. It is the prime agent that stops fatty acids from reacting with oxygen to form harmful toxins known as lipid peroxides. Vitamin E is necessary for the health of the reproductive system, the integrity of red blood cells and for the functioning of the white blood cells of the immune system.

Vitamin C is the 'goes everywhere, does everything' nutrient. If you choose to take a single vitamin supplement, vitamin C would be a prime candidate, as it is involved in so many different parts of the body, from the immune system to the connective tissue that literally holds us together. Vitamin C is not manufactured in the body, so to maintain health we must acquire adequate vitamin C supplies from our diet.

More vitamin C is required when we are in demanding situations since it is involved in the production of adrenaline, our 'fight or flight' hormone; it is itself consumed, acting as an anti-oxidant, and it is vital for tissue and bone growth and repair. Its effect on specific parts of the protective immune system include the modulation of the action of white blood cells, a fact that has excited researchers such as Nobel Prize winner Linus Pauling. It may even be linked to the natural production of Interferon.

We depend on vitamin C to produce collagen, the structural protein that holds our cells together and is an integral part of skin, tendons, bone cartilages, and the other connective tissues that package our muscles and organs. Vitamin C is important for healthy bones and, in particular, for healthy teeth and gums, as it combines with minerals such as calcium and phosphorus.

Iron, the red blood cell mineral, is better absorbed in the presence of vitamin C, while the proper functioning of other nutrients, such as selenium and vitamins A and E, also depends on adequate vitamin C. It also supports vitamin E in its role of protecting fatty acids from harmful oxidation.

Although we need a regular and dependable intake of vitamin C in food, it is highly vulnerable to heat and light and can be almost entirely lost if food is incorrectly stored or cooked. It is an interesting fact that gorillas, who, like us, 'lost' the ability to manufacture vitamin C during evolution, take in upwards of three grammes of vitamin C each day.

Unlike us, they still live surrounded by plentiful supplies of vitamin C-rich fresh vegetation and fruit, and they eat it raw.

The single most important source of vitamin C in the British diet is the potato. When potatoes are chipped and fried, a lot of vitamin C is lost. In addition, it is thought that our vitamin C requirements fluctuate, not only according to biochemical individuality, but also because of what is going on in our lives. At particular times our needs increase. Being water soluble, vitamin C is quickly transported through the body and excreted, mainly in urine, and therefore regular replenishing is advisable.

People who use drugs, such as aspirin, antibiotics and the contraceptive pill, quite wisely often choose to take vitamin C supplements, as do regular alcohol drinkers and smokers. Other groups who may benefit from a supplement are athletes in training, the elderly and pregnant, and breast-feeding women.

Recognising its importance as a nutrient, Nature's Best produce twenty-two different vitamin C supplements in order to cater for differences in individual requirements and Nature's Best were the pioneers of the easy-to-use powder form of sodium- or calcium-buffered version of vitamin C and the development of vitamin C in crystals, powder, time-release tablets, and capsules has made them UK leaders in vitamin C technology. They have also introduced a fat soluble form to widen its anti-oxidant capabilities.

8

Parasitic Infections

I REMEMBER clearly, when I was still quite young, my first encounter with *parasitic infections*, although at the time the word meant nothing to me. We were awakened in the middle of the night by the doorbell. A caller at that time of the night is most unusual at any time, but this was during the war years, so we were especially wary. Half-curious and half-frightened I crept behind my mother when she opened the door and outside stood a man wearing a shoe on one foot and a clog on the other. At that time my mother had people hidden in our house from the Germans, and when our visitor told her that he had escaped from one of the ships that would have taken him on his way to a concentration camp in Germany, she quickly pulled him inside. His presence in the house endangered all our lives but, at least inside he had a measure of safety, certainly more so than walking the streets. My mother, however, was faced with a considerable dilemma. She soon discovered that it would be irresponsible to let him mix with the other people in hiding, because our latest guest had *scabies*. This condition was more common during the war years, and it was fortunate that my mother, although not professionally trained, was very knowledgeable about homoeopathic and naturopathic remedies. She explained that if the house were to be searched she could not let him hide under the floor with the others because of the infectiousness of his condition, and she would have to treat him. The man was covered from top to toe in ointment, so that, if need be, he could also hide out in the space cleared under the floor.

Scabies is a highly contagious, parasitic skin disease, and its many eruptions cause intense itching. It is caused by the so-called itch mite and I have been told that it is enough to drive one mad. The treatment is basically external and sulphur echtiol, the cream used by my mother, is one of the best methods for treating a person with this disease. However, as the itch can become unbearable, it may be necessary to prescribe something for internal use as well. I have great faith in the Bioforce remedy, Boldocynara, which helps to ease the itching condition. This remedy is a fresh herbal preparation and should be taken three times a day, ten to fifteen drops in a little water. It contains the following ingredients:

Artichoke	St Mary's Thistle
Knotweed	Dandelion
Boldo	Barberry
Radish	Peppermint
Aloe	Club Moss

Another parasitic infection, fortunately less and less common nowadays, is *Pediculosis*, which is also a lice infestation. This condition was also common during the war years and I remember that eventually we just shrugged our shoulders when, at school, we heard that someone would be absent for a few days because that usually meant they had been infested with lice and taken into hospital. Yet, prior to the war and since, there was a tremendous stigma attached to such conditions.

The *Pediculus capitis*, a head louse, is usually limited to the scalp, while the *Pediculus corporis* inhabits the seams of clothing worn next to the skin, and feeds on the skin covered by clothes. Usually the condition can be treated externally, but if it is persistent internal treatment may also be necessary. In days gone by, the old-fashioned remedy DDT was often used. Nowadays it is recognised that this poisonous substance can have very considerable after-effects. Although it was effective, there are natural treatment methods that are equally good, e.g. stinging nettle extract.

There are some very good ointments available for scabious conditions, one of which is a garlic ointment. Although smelly, it is quite effective, even for the condition of *Pediculosis pubis*, where the crab louse infests the hairs of the genital region. Occasionally it is also found in the eyebrows, eyelashes, beard or sometimes on the body surface.

These conditions are extremely unpleasant and socially embarrassing. Thanks to better hygiene standards, these conditions are nowhere near as common as they were during the traumatic war years. However, if they do occur, immediate treatment should be sought.

9

Yeast Infections

I WAS quite tempted to call this chapter *Yeast and Wheat Infections*, as the two very often go hand in hand. The reader may wonder if there really is such a thing as a 'wheat infection'. Indeed there is, and it is actually a relatively common occurrence. I see so many patients, who come to me as a last resort after they have seen doctors and skin specialists, and yet have not seen any improvement in their skin problems. Often they come to me with the news that according to their doctor or specialist they have an 'unidentified skin disorder'. Frequently, the first thing I do is advise the patient to immediately leave out wheat and yeast from the diet.

Once wheat was considered a major constituent of man's staple diet. In modern days, due to artificial fertilising, herbicides and pesticides, it sometimes does not even deserve to be part of our diet at all. In their earliest forms, wheat grains contained four chromosomes. Now the average wheat grain contains sixty, seventy or even more chromosomes, as a result of our methods of fertilisation. My book *Viruses, Allergies and the Immune System* contains a chapter entitled *Nutrition and Mental Behaviour* which deals in considerable detail with this subject. In that chapter I wrote about patients whose brains were unable to cope with all these chromosomes and their diets had to reflect limitation.

Wheat is also responsible for the fungus *Candida albicans* and although there is ever more information on this condition and its cause, it nevertheless seems to be spreading steadily. This yeast parasite can be very persistent, and the problems caused by the candida are not only visible on the skin, but may also be present in the intestines, vagina and mouth. Micro-organisms, yeast and bacteria, inhabit the gut where a very delicate balance reigns, and an irritable bowel syndrome is sometimes an indication of a candida infection. Yet, these signs are not often correctly interpreted. Another way still for a candida to make its presence known is a deterioration in skin condition while taking antibiotics. It isn't only the skin that is affected; often the patient experiences unusual food cravings, diarrhoea, a bloated feeling, intestinal wind, constant tiredness, weight gain and depression. These symptoms combine to weaken the immune system, allowing the yeast infection to become a very real problem. Under these circumstances homoeopathy probably presents more treatment options than allopathic medicine. Unfortunately, a candidiasis too often remains undetected until the person concerned experiences persistent skin irritations, itchings and recurrent bouts of vaginal irritation. Anal irritation is another frequent symptom.

The occurrence of *Candida albicans* is largely due to our dietary habits. It can easily be called a twentieth-century disease, because our lifestyle and environment allow allergies more and more opportunities to develop. Yeast is naturally present in everyone from the age of about six months. The risk of candida infections is greatly reduced by a natural, balanced diet.

In a lecture given by Dr Alfred Vogel quite some time ago, he spoke about friendly bacteria in the bowels which are frequently killed off by the food we eat. One wouldn't think that asking a patient to change his or her diet would be too much of an imposition, but this suggestion isn't always enthusiastically received. Sometimes I think that people have less trouble changing their religion, their political allegiance, or even their husband or wife, than changing their diet. All I ask is that they cut five foods from their diet, namely sugar, mushrooms, wine, fermented foods or drinks, and chocolate. When I mention sugary foods, I mean all foods that contain sugar. Of the fermented foods, bread is probably the most difficult one to replace. Most alcoholic drinks are fermented and are therefore off limits. Only by following these guidelines, and by introducing a natural diet with lots of vegetables, fruits and nuts, and drinking plenty of water, do we have a chance of combating a candida problem successfully.

The discovery of antibiotics was quite rightly hailed as a tremendous discovery and many lives have since been saved. Yet, the word antibiotic actually means 'anti-life' and unfortunately antibiotics are not selective in the bacteria they destroy. Often the good or friendly bacteria are killed off along with the harmful bacteria. It is these friendly bacteria we rely upon for digestion and for our general good health. Control and balance of a candida is very important and fortunately there are several good remedies that will assist us in this. Harpagophytum (Devil's Claw extract in its mother tincture) is one of the best remedies to control a *candida* or yeast infection. Molkosan may be used and Caprylic acid, a derivative of coconut oil, has also been used successfully, especially when the candida is active in the vaginal area.

Deficiency of essential fatty acids may also result in a greater likelihood of developing a candida infection. These acids contain Omega three and Omega six, essential to health. There are three 'essential' fatty acids: linoleic, arachidonic, and linolenic, collectively known as vitamin F. They are termed 'essential' because the body cannot produce them. These unsaturated fatty acids are necessary for growth and healthy blood, arteries and nerves. They also help to keep the skin and other tissues youthful and healthy by preventing dryness and scaliness. Essential fatty acids are necessary too for the transport and breakdown of cholesterol. Evening primrose oil, borage oil and blackcurrant seed oil are all good sources of essential fatty acids, and these oils change as we react to the environment with respect to the cell membranes. There are also some oils that are actually detrimental from this point of view, such as peanut oil and coconut oil. The body tissues are made of what we eat, and how we respond to our environment depends totally on how strong the tissues are. Life is a constant renewal of cell tissue and in order to rebuild tissue we need the correct material. Topically applied and absorbed fatty acids can be of great help here, even for babies with skin problems. Even a very young baby can change metabolically when the right oils are used and will improve very quickly.

If the diet is poor, supplementary Omega three and six tend to produce a more anti-inflammatory response. Skin irritation or injury will cause the cells to go into a coagulation response, stimulating the reaction of white blood cells and increasing the production of leucotrines. This can be clearly seen in the skin condition *psoriasis*. The more leucotrines or inflammatory response, the more division and proliferation of cells is necessary to decrease this reaction. One of the remedies that can be very useful here is Ginkgo biloba.

Ginkgo biloba is the world's oldest living tree species. Its lineage stretches back 200 million years, and although it originated in China, it grows to a ripe old age in the many other parts of the world to which it has been transplanted. Modern scientific analysis has revealed the reason Ginkgo trees have survived for so long: their leaves are packed with highly-active chemicals that give the tree unusual resistance to parasites, infections and pollution. The leaves of the

Ginkgo are traditionally harvested in the autumn, just as the colour changes, and this is exactly the time when they have their highest active concentrations of bioflavonoids. These are now thought to be most potent of all bioflavonoids, and are thought to have the ability to help maintain the circulation of blood to the brain.

To increase the Omega three factor, flax seed, cod liver and sunflower oil are helpful, as well as selenium and betacarotene. A combination of vitamin E with flax seed oil is totally suitable for the treatment of this affliction. Linoleic acid production is helped by biotin, magnesium, vitamin B_6 and zinc. Unfortunately this is obstructed by the use of alcohol, high cholesterol foods, saturated fats, virus infections, and cancer. Evening primrose oil helps to form DGLA (dihomo gammalinolenic acid), which in turn needs vitamin B_3, vitamin C and extra zinc to form prostaglandins, necessary in the case of all skin disorders.

Many skin disorders are self-inflicted insofar as they are the result of modern dietary habits. The many patients with yeast infections I have been asked to treat over the years have all been greatly helped when nutritional deficiencies have been dealt with, together with some herbal or homoeopathic treatment. Evening primrose oil, sometimes in combination with fish oil, has been of great help, as well as vitamin A and C supplements.

In countries where the wheat intake is low I have never seen an active *candidiasis*, which leads me to believe that our lifestyle, wheat consumption and the number of processed food items in our diet, all have a great deal to answer for. Organically-grown wheat is much less harmful, but, if a definite wheat allergy has been proven, it must be banned from the diet. If the candida albicans condition is indeed affecting the vaginal and anal areas, dabbing with some diluted Molkosan will ease the discomfort, and sometimes it is useful to know that the skin will soften with witch hazel (*Hamamelis virginiana*). The Bioforce range also has a witch hazel cream, called Hamamelis salve, which also contains St John's Wort, echinacea and wheat germ oil.

Patients are not always prepared to accept changes in their diet, and I often have to explain that, even if they are not willing to accept a major change of direction, the very least they ought to do is leave out sugar and hopefully yeast. Just eliminating these substances often brings about a considerable change. I often wonder why people suffer such unpleasant problems, when they can be helped so easily. Never underestimate a yeast infection, because it is likely to lead to greater problems if it goes unchecked. In research, active candida conditions have been found in cancer patients and, together with this word of warning, I also want to encourage the sufferer that yeast infections and *Candida albicans* can be treated successfully. However, never delay seeking help when the condition comes to light.

10

Pellagra

IT IS several years now since I wrote my first book *Stress and Nervous Disorders*. I remember writing about a young lady who came to see me in one of my clinics in the South of England. The lady was upset and very tense as she had been diagnosed and classified as mentally unstable. Yet when I spoke to her, I felt doubtful about this conclusion and it soon became clear that she suffered from a condition called *pellagra*, which, by her own admission, made her impossible to live with. Pellagra is described as a chronic disease, caused by a deficiency of niacin in the diet, and characterised by skin eruptions and mental disorders. It is the label of mental illness that is most difficult to shake. I still see her occasionally, and there is little that reminds me of the person who, so many years ago, walked into my consulting rooms. This metamorphosis is largely due to the fact that she no longer suffers from pellagra.

When I first interviewed her, she told me that she had

been on a weight-reducing diet and that she had taken appetite-suppressing drugs. She had indeed managed to lose a considerable amount of weight and she also told me that she remembered feeling very clear in her mind. At no time did she ever consider the idea that she might be suffering from malnutrition. Although she thought that the diet and resulting weight loss had done her a lot of good, after a while the first signs appeared of her brain and nerve cells having suffered from lack of nutrition.

As soon as I saw her I recognised her skin problem as pellagra and I told her that her only way to recover was to follow a healthy and balanced diet. I reassured her that if she kept to the instructions she need not worry about regaining any of the weight she had shed with such effort. In fact it was largely due to her weight loss that she had become deficient in the B Complex vitamins, and therefore I immediately prescribed vitamin B_6 and vitamin C.

It is not unusual for vitamin deficiencies to occur when diets become unbalanced and sometimes this is the case, even with carefully worked out slimming diets. In these cases I always introduce a diet rich in soya and rice, as these are valuable dietary supplements. With supplementary minerals such as potassium, chromium, selenium and the B vitamins, many deficiencies can be redressed. Once I had explained to this patient the basis of my diagnosis and resulting recommendations, she was as conscientious in following my dietary instructions as she had been when she wanted to lose weight. She soon noticed a remarkable improvement in the condition of her skin. Some Niacin and vitamin B_3 gave her a little extra help and the end results took her by surprise.

With a long-standing problem like pellagra, it is essential to rebuild the body. Once the diagnosis has been reached, some remedies or supplements can be introduced, including oil of evening primrose and additional vitamins, minerals and trace elements. Given today's harassed and frantic life-style, the B vitamins are vital. They are particularly important for the health of nerves and the brain, and also for defence against infections. As man is not able to store B vitamins, we must ensure a ready supply in our diet. Moreover, B vitamins are water soluble and therefore easily lost in the cooking process. This information should be kept in mind when deciding on a vitamin supplement.

When advising a patient to use a B Complex supplement I usually recommend Vitamin B-Complex from Nature's Best, for its balanced composition and use of natural sources. One capsule a day provides:

Vitamin B_1 (Thiamin)	10 mg	Folic Acid	400 mcg
Vitamin B_2 (Riboflavin)	10 mg	Biotin	100 mcg
Vitamin B_6 (Pyridoxine		PABA	20 mg
Hydrochloride)	10 mg	Pangamic Acid	30 mg
Vitamin B_{12}	10 mcg	Choline	150 mg
Pantothenic Acid	80 mg	Inositol	150 mg
Nicotinamide	60 mg	Vitamin C	100 mg

Taking a vitamin B Complex supplement to correct vitamin deficiencies, will maintain the nerves and the nervous system in good order, release energy from our carbohydrate fuel, maintain the health of our digestive tract, repair and regenerate the circulatory system, assist the metabolic process of fats and proteins, and maintain healthy eyes, hair, skin and mucous membranes.

Especially in the case of a pellagra condition, it is worth noting that after taking vitamin B_3 or Niacin, if the vitamin is taken in its nicotinic acid form, a flushing or tingling sensation can sometimes be experienced. It is often also considered necessary to take vitamin B_2 or Riboflavin which is one of the co-enzymes which enables us to utilise oxygen safely and effectively. It is involved in the conversion of protein, fats and sugar into energy. It is important for the eyes, skin, hair and nails, and for the repair and maintenance of soft tissue, such as the lips, tongue, and mucous membranes in the mouth (for example). Again this vitamin is water soluble and therefore not stored in large amounts and must be regularly provided in the diet. Since the richest food sources of Riboflavin include liver and yeast, vegetarians often choose to take a vitamin B_2 supplement. Riboflavin naturally has a strong yellow colour and sometimes is the cause of highly-coloured urine, but it is harmless.

If the skin has suffered for a long period of time from a pellagra condition, it is possible to introduce some remedies to help restore good health. Again, I feel that the natural herbal antibiotic, Echinaforce, is of great help. Another symptom of pellagra can be unpleasant gastro-intestinal complaints. In these cases the Centaurium (corn flower) remedy should be used and this can be easily combined with Echinaforce and the vitamin supplements.

Many skin conditions are the result of dietary habits and the more white sugar, fats and animal protein our diet contains, the smaller the reserves of certain vitamins, and this most definitely includes Niacin. This vitamin also plays a major part in cholesterol problems and if the skin is blemished, as it can be with cholesterol deposits, Niacin will help to put this right. We sometimes overlook the fact that our food does not contain the nutrients it used to, and vitamin supplements are therefore increasingly necessary.

The definition of 'vitamin' is an organic food substance, essential for the normal metabolism of other nutrients, the promotion of growth and the maintenance of health. Not all vitamins can be synthesised within the body. Vitamins are essential for regulating the metabolism, they help to convert fat and carbohydrates into energy, and they assist in the formation, growth and repair of bone tissue. Vitamins are also essential for reproduction, formation of antibodies, coagulation of blood, formulation of intercellular substances, and for the integrity of bone, skin, blood and nervous tissue. They function as co-enzymes for innumerable chemical reactions concerned with the metabolism of food on which the nutrition of the body really depends. It is also true that essential micro-nutrients, or metabolic activators, have a specific activity in the prevention of deficiency diseases and that the same nutrients are important to life's process.

11

Pityriasis Rosea

PITYRIASIS ROSEA is an acute inflammatory disease of the skin with severe scaling and flaking of the outer layer, often in circular patches. The cause appears to be unknown, although it is thought to be the result of a viral agent. This skin disorder affects both male and female, producing low-grade fever and headaches. A further symptom is that it can cause moments of real distress prior to the occurrence of the skin eruptions. Fortunately the lesions do not often appear on the facial skin, but when present they display themselves mostly on the palms of the hands and the soles of the feet. These can become very dry and cause cracks, coupled with intense skin irritation. It is possible that the problem may burn itself out, but it is better not to take a chance and to seek medical advice. Usually this condition responds well to Echinaforce, the natural antibiotic from the Bioforce range. As pityriasis rosea is relatively uncommon, it sometimes takes a little time before it is diagnosed correctly.

In some pityriasis rosea patients I have found that the thyroid gland was either under- or over-active. (It is commonly observed that skin disorders often involve the thyroid gland.) Usually this indicates a hormonal imbalance, or a deficiency of essential fatty acids. Sometimes I suggest that the body temperature is measured ten minutes before getting out of bed in the morning, by placing a thermometer under the arm. If the temperature is under 36.5 degrees Celsius, it could well be that the thyroid is under-active and this must be brought to the attention of a doctor or practitioner. With an over-active thyroid, the temperature is usually over 36.8 degrees Celsius, and medical treatment may also be necessary.

As with most skin disorders, I would prescribe vitamin F. Lecithin is a better-known name for this vitamin, although this is not quite correct as vitamin F mostly appears in unsaturated fatty acids. Vitamin F helps to regulate the rate of blood coagulation and performs a vital function in breaking up cholesterol deposited on arterial walls. It is essential for normal glandular activity, especially of the adrenal glands and the thyroid gland, and it also nourishes the skin and is essential for healthy mucous membranes and nerves. It can be of great help when combined with Lecithin. Deficiency of vitamin F can lead to a raised metabolic rate and frequently displays itself externally as eczema. As vitamin F is in short supply in most diets, it is well worth knowing the foods that are rich in this vitamin, i.e. soya beans, soya oil, sunflower, corn and wheat germ oil, and oily fish, such as salmon, tuna, halibut, and mackerel. For many skin conditions I recommend rice, which is an excellent balanced food and rich in vitamin F. Eating nuts such as almonds and brazils can also be helpful as these contain a great deal of vitamin F. Over-activity of the sebaceous glands is restricted by vitamin F which explains its relevance to the thyroid glands. The combined vitamins E and F perform an excellent task in most skin conditions, but especially so in the case of pityriasis rosea. Among homoeopathic remedies, I must single out phosphorus.

A while ago, a Jamaican lady who thought that she had pityriasis rosea came to see me. When I studied her skin I noticed some similarities, but I wasn't quite convinced. It transpired that she suffered from a condition called *Lupus erythematosus*, a condition I have also written about in my book *Arthritis, Rheumatism and Psoriasis*. The *lupus* condition, however, is ten times worse than pityriasis, and certainly requires specialised medical attention. This lady told me that she had been advised to use extract of couch grass, which is a marvellous kidney cleanser and therefore of great help, especially for lupus conditions. However, for pityriasis rosea I prefer to use Harpagophytum, and advise patients to brew this as a tea, which can be drunk in small amounts several times during the day. If the condition is very persistent I also recommend Petasan (extract of the petasites root). A mixture of herbal tea made from catnip, bayberry, golden seal, myrrh, Irish moss, fenugreek, chickweed, comfrey root, cayenne, buckle weed and yellow dog, will help to overcome this condition very quickly.

Earlier I mentioned the use of garlic (although I can understand that people have objections to the lingering smell). Fortunately Nature's Best have produced Pure-Gar, a deodorised garlic capsule. The medicinal use of garlic is cheap when compared to the price of drugs and as garlic has a host of medicinal qualities, not only for culinary and internal use, but also for the treatment of wounds or as an antiseptic, I can well understand why people have such a high regard for this wonderful remedy which grows freely in the wild. Garlic is one of the few foods that contain vitamin B_{17}, which is the anti-cancer vitamin. It has many other properties because it activates not only the glands, but will restore the bacterial balance in the bowels and cleanse the blood. It is therefore useful for angina and circulatory and skin problems.

For pityriasis rosea I would also like to add some dietary

guidelines. For a period of time eliminate all meat and fish from the diet, and white flour, white sugar, fried foods, coffee, sweets, chocolate and alcohol. Instead eat lots of raw fruits and vegetables and wholemeal bread. Avoid stress and take action to ensure that the system is free of constipation. Activate the skin by sunbathing and try some hydrotherapy treatment: alternate the bath water from hot to cold and change from a shower to the bath.

For external use I would recommend St John's Wort Oil from Dr Vogel, or dab the affected skin areas with PoHo oil or linseed oil. At all costs I would advise avoiding steroid creams or other strong ointments or creams. Use instead the Seven Herb Cream, Bioforce Cream or Echinacea Cream. These creams are all readily absorbed into the skin and this allows the active ingredients in the herbal extract to begin working immediately, without leaving an oily residue.

It used to be thought that it was impossible for creams to be absorbed by the skin. This was because the skin, and especially the outer layer, or epidermis, acts as a barrier and makes it impossible for water to penetrate the skin. This is quite logical, considering that one of the most important functions of the skin is to protect the body against external influences. Under an electron microscope it is possible to count nineteen layers that together make up the epidermis. These layers consist of flattened, dead cells which are closely packed together. Between these cells, lipids can be found which act as a glue-like substance. Tiny glands in the skin secrete a fatty substance, for the purpose of destroying bacteria on the surface, which explains the general assumption that the skin can neither absorb nor be penetrated. Modern technological research, however, has found ways of penetrating the skin. Firstly, skin penetration can be influenced positively by good skin care and cleanliness. Secondly, medical research has revealed the presence of liposomes, which are sometimes described as minute 'transport balls or bubbles'. Since then this knowledge has been used to great advantage by the cosmetics industry. It is the minute size of the liposomes that allows them to penetrate the skin, both through the cells and in between the cells of the epidermis. It is thanks to this relatively new technology that we can now happily recommend such treatment creams as those mentioned above for the benefit of skin conditions.

12

Vitiligo

THE OTHER DAY I was visited by a distinguished, well-dressed gentleman, who told me that he was prepared to undergo any treatment in order to be cured of his skin condition. He had been diagnosed as suffering from a condition called *vitiligo*, a skin disease characterised by pigment-free patches surrounded by a darker band, which can occur anywhere on the body. Hairs that grow on these patches of skin are colourless and the condition originates from a melanin disturbance. The gentleman explained that he was sometimes ashamed even to offer to shake hands, as the vitiligo condition was very visible on his upper limbs. (The skin affliction on other parts of his body was naturally not quite as obvious.)

I immediately recognised the condition, because I have come across it often in Asian people who have emigrated to the United Kingdom. I can well understand that it is a cause of embarrassment to people, but the condition can be helped and although loss of pigmentation causes the milky-white patches surrounded by hyper pigmented borders, the tissue of the skin is otherwise unaltered.

Officially the cause of vitiligo is unknown, but over the years I have reached the conclusion that it is nutrition-related. This premise has resulted in an individual treatment approach which has proven relatively successful. Another unfortunate characteristic is that usually these pigment-free patches increase quickly, and therefore it is very hard to attempt to cover the affected areas of the skin with make-up.

The gentleman in question was reasonably successful in blocking the development of new patches with special skin brushing methods. He also used cold water treatments and a variety of herbs, e.g. burdock, chaparral, oregon, coke-wood, and red clover blossom. I also prescribed Chelidonium, which he used in a homoeopathic form to help the skin in general. At a lecture, I had heard that a deficiency of zinc can influence the condition and quality of the skin, and therefore I also advised him to use a zinc supplement.

According to leading nutrition researchers, such as Dr Carl Pfeiffer, people find it more difficult to obtain enough zinc than any other mineral. Soil deficiencies of zinc have reduced levels available in plant foods, and zinc is removed by food processing. High levels of calcium and phosphates found in plant foods or fertilisers are thought to block absorption of zinc from food. The body's stores of zinc may be threatened by missing meals, weight-reducing diets or fasting. The most reliable sources of zinc are shellfish, herrings and meat, and many vegetarians choose to supplement their diet with zinc. Smokers, alcohol drinkers, users of the contraceptive pill, the elderly, and athletes (zinc is lost in perspiration) may also take extra zinc.

Zinc is well known for its role in growth and tissue repair and in the immune system. It is vital that children and adolescents receive enough. Zinc is not only required for overall growth, but it is particularly important for the healthy function of reproductive organs and the prostate gland. It is also a component of semen. But these functions only scratch the surface of zinc's importance, since it is involved in hundreds of metabolic pathways. Some of these maintain vision and our senses of smell and taste; others deal with digestion of carbohydrates and the balance of blood-sugar controlling insulin, the absorption of other nutrients, such as vitamin A and the B-complex vitamins, and cell metabolism. It is so important because it is a part of many different chemical catalysts, or enzymes. It is also one of our most important antioxidants, as part of the major antioxidant enzyme, super-oxide dismutase (SOD), and protects cells from the damage caused by oxidising fats.

Nature's Best has led the way by making high-quality zinc supplements available. The first manufacturer to offer an inexpensive and reliable taste-testing kit, Nature's Best has also been quick to use new technology to make available new forms of zinc supplements. A breakthrough that is still popular, not just in winter, is the convenient, orange-flavoured Zinc-Plus Lozenge.

I have also noticed with vitiligo sufferers, especially in the Asian community, that many are often very thirsty. It is quite possible that the liver also plays a small part in this condition, and the body reacts as if it does not have enough fluids. First the secretions of the glands are reduced and saliva dries up, indications that the level of body fluids is too low. Body fluids provide the internal environment for the billions of body cells which constitute up to 55 or 60 per cent of total body weight. In addition to serving as the fluid conveyor of nutrients, body fluids are used as a route for removal of waste. The intake of water, to maintain balance, should equal the output. Fluid intake takes place from all kinds of food and drink: loss of fluid includes a fixed loss through the lungs, perspiration and a variable loss through the kidneys. Extra-cellular fluid, or that outside of the cells, makes up 35 per cent of the total. All extra-cellular fluids are nearly identical in type and concentration, but differ in protein concentration. Sodium and chloride are the primary extra-cellular electrolytes, while protein concentration is highest in plasma compartments. Intra-cellular fluid contains more protein than extra-cellular fluid and contains potassium and phosphate as primary electrolytes.

Electrolytes are electrically charged particles, ions that conduct electricity. Amino acids act as transporters to conduct these charged particles through membranes. Electrolytes are needed in order to establish osmosis (which is the movement between cell walls from areas of high to low density, the balancing nutrients), as components in buffer systems and in the acceptability in all cells of membrane potentials. The principal electrolytes with a positive charge are sodium, potassium, calcium and magnesium. Electrolytes with a negative charge are chloride, phosphate, sulphate and bicarbonate.

I have described the behaviour of fluids and the body balance in detail in order to demonstrate that fluids are essential for purification of the system and, ultimately, the skin. Better balance here often causes vitiligo to reduce or even disappear. It was very satisfying to notice a steady improvement in the condition of the gentleman I mentioned earlier. I have treated quite a number of vitiligo patients, some with good results and others with no change at all. There is certainly no easy treatment; for instance I have discovered that it cannot be cured by sunshine. However, drinking ginseng and chamomile tea sometimes helps and I usually advise that the patient does so three times daily. Dietary instructions are to avoid acid-containing foods, e.g. pork, sweet foods, coffee, tea, and chocolate. Whether these foods are detrimental to the development of vitiligo is not certain, but I am in no doubt that they will definitely not help to overcome this embarrassing skin condition.

13

Lichen Planus

IN MORE than thirty years of practice I have never come across as many cases of *Lichen planus* as recently. Although it is by no means a common problem, I am concerned at the increased incidence of this particular skin disorder. Lichen planus is an inflammatory dermatosis which manifests itself in multiple, small, flat-topped patches, with a reddish colour and a horny appearance. This skin disorder affects both sexes, and it is quite likely that its greater incidence is due to increased stress, anxiety and nervous disorders. If not the actual causes of this disease, they are more than likely to be serious contributory factors. Although this condition can be short-lived, I have also seen chronic cases, which are very difficult to overcome once they have been allowed to establish themselves. There is a general belief that improper nutrition and insomnia are also possible factors that aggravate this condition.

Initially I would choose to treat the nervous system and,

for this purpose, I would suggest breathing exercises, which exert a relaxing influence. The 'Hara Breathing Exercise', explained in detail in my book *Stress and Nervous Disorders*, is of great help, as are a number of exercises that encourage relaxation. Treatments that produce good perspiration are also helpful. For this reason Turkish baths and saunas are suggested, since they are relaxing, at the same time as encouraging perspiration. When taking a sauna, the temperature of the entire skin increases to between 40 and 43 degrees Celsius. This increase in temperature intensifies the circulation while the increase in perspiration stimulates cell renewal and can eliminate some 20 to 30 grammes of fluid per minute from the body. Showering with cold water and warm foot baths causes the pores to open and the blood vessels to widen, which gives these bathing methods therapeutic value.

It is also a good idea to do some breathing exercises while taking a sauna, as the circulation through the lungs and air passages is excellent at high temperatures. At any time, go out into the fresh air and inhale deeply to fill the lungs with oxygen, thus stimulating the sympathetic nervous system. Due to increased hormone production, stress will be reduced when taking a regular sauna. Centuries ago in Finland, when the sauna was no more than a hole in the ground with some heated stones, saunas were recognised for their therapeutic value. Even though a sauna is taken under more luxurious conditions nowadays, that therapeutic value has not diminished, but take care not to stay in a sauna for too long. It is better to increase the frequency of saunas, with a good rest period in between, than to take occasional saunas for a long time, which may be unwise. I often advise that a first sauna should not be longer than eight to twelve minutes, with a cooling-off period of about the same length of time. During this time apply some Kneipp methods and use a good body spray. Have a warm foot bath and, if accompanied, joining in a conversation will aid relaxation. If possible, try some sunray treatment, but better still if it is possible, go outside to enjoy the sun: any ultra-violet treatment after a sauna course will be of great help for a lichen planus condition.

Infra-red treatment on the affected areas is also beneficial, but mostly I prefer ultra-violet treatment, because under the influence of ultra-violet rays, substances such as ergosterin are converted into vitamin D which is of great benefit to the overall condition of the skin.

From time to time a skin brushing session is helpful. Use a natural brush and allow twenty to thirty minutes to brush every part of the body that is not affected by *lichen planus*, remembering always to brush towards the heart. It is best to start with the soles of the feet and a dry body. Brush the skin surface with regular movements, avoiding any affected areas, the face, and genital areas. Use clean, upward-sweeping strokes remembering that below the heart all brushing movement should be upwards, while over the heart downward strokes only. Use light and gentle pressure and perhaps a herbal ointment or a herbal oil afterwards, e.g. Symphosan, lemon or orange oil from the Bioforce range. Another remedy from the same source, Petasan, should be taken three times a day, ten drops after meals, and to encourage quick healing, use evening primrose oil and Violaforce. This is the best possible advice to get a *lichen planus* condition under control.

Because of the influence of stress on this skin condition, I sometimes recommend a juice diet, or even a fasting regime allowing fruit and vegetable juices only. However, I would advise excluding citrus fruit juices in such a regime. A period of fasting will be beneficial to most of the body's systems and functions, such as digestion, blood circulation, elimination from the bowels and kidneys, nerve vitality, respiration and oxygenation. I recommend fasting courses for diverse purposes, but especially for lichen planus as so many bodily functions and systems are affected by it.

On the first day of a fast there might be some slight discomfort, but a few days of fasting will be extremely beneficial. Better still, if after an initial period of fasting, one selects a specific day of the week on which to fast on a regular basis. Fasting allows the body to rid itself of some of the many toxins that are present, and you will soon recognise the feeling of well-being that takes over after one or more days. Don't worry if you experience a slight dull headache, because this often occurs when the tissues eliminate toxins, which are disposed of into the bloodstream and work their way to the head.

Many patients report a feeling of cleanliness (inside as well as out) after fasting and most repeat the experience. Simply replace meals with a drink of vegetable or fruit juice. The age-old naturopathic principle that an occasional period of fasting is beneficial, has never held more truth and wisdom than at present.

14

Psoriasis

I HAVE purposely left *psoriasis* for the last chapter, as I am well aware that one could fill an entire book on the subject. The key question is whether or not there is a cure for psoriasis and I am happy to say that I have seen quite a number of psoriasis patients who can claim full recovery. Although psoriasis is a chronic skin disease which causes a great deal of distress, it can often be overcome, but this requires perseverence and a positive frame of mind.

Once again I should stress that the skin condition reflects conditions inside the body, and therefore a naturopathic approach will serve the patient much better than layers of cortisone or tar ointment plastered over the skin, since this deals only in part with the symptoms, while the actual cause of the problem remains present inside the body. Psoriasis ought to be treated internally and to this end, a diet to establish an acid/alkaline balance in the body is essential. Such a diet has been described in one of my previous books

Arthritis, Rheumatism and Psoriasis, and I still maintain that this is the correct foundation on which to develop a programme for psoriasis treatment.

Psoriasis is often compared to arthritis, in which case it is referred to as *psoriatica arthritica*, but there are many kinds of psoriasis. This chronic inflammatory skin disease lasts for several years and has been the cause of concern and unhappiness for many people. Although it is generally believed that the cause of psoriasis is unknown, in my experience it is definitely largely diet related. With many of my patients I have seen, that if they are prepared to follow dietary instructions, the condition will clear. Unfortunately it is impossible to predict how long the treatment period will be, because the rate of improvement varies greatly among patients. I sympathise with the many people who suffer from this disease and their plight has challenged me to do everything within my power to help them. The worst possible attitude is that one 'will have to learn to live with it'. No health problem must be allowed to linger and this is never more true than in the case of psoriasis.

One of the most troublesome conditions is known as *mother of pearl scales*, where flaking skin peels off, leaving a shiny surface, sometimes so thin that blood seems to be visible immediately under the surface. These patches can be quite large and may appear anywhere on the body; it is not unusual for nails and/or joints to be affected. Although this skin condition does not appear to affect one's health, it can cause considerable stiffness when it is related to arthritis. It is also a great cause of embarrassment and therefore Hahnemann's principle is important: to treat mind, body and spirit. Nothing is gained by sitting back and wallowing in self-pity, because one gets more uptight and more nervous, which in turn aggravates the psoriatic condition, causing it to spread further and become more angry and deep-rooted. Many psoriasis patients will agree with me that they have periods when they seem to be able to cope reasonably well, until they pass through a stressful phase, and it's then that the skin condition will suddenly flare up again.

So, what are the treatment options for psoriasis? Well, the first requirement must be to ensure that internally the body is in a sufficiently good condition to allow healing to start. This means that the basic condition for effective psoriasis treatment is a balanced diet. For many years my patients have had a high rate of success with the following diet, where a choice can be made between items listed under each section.

Breakfast:
Compote of stewed apple, dates, blackberries and prunes.
Mixture of dates, apple and blackberries.
Porridge sweetened with molasses or honey, and soya milk or prune juice only.
Brown rice and/or barley (cooked) served with soya sauce or stewed apple.
Rye crispbread.

Lunch:
Salad of any raw vegetables except tomatoes or peppers. Raw apple, grated carrots, onions and garlic, cress and alfalfa seed sprouts are especially good in a salad.
Four to eight ounces of grated carrots every day for carotene.
Blended vegetable soup with Plantaforce used for stock.
Two slices of rye crispbread or one slice of pumpernickel bread.
Jacket potato, brown rice and/or barley, millet, or millet and potato.

Dinner:
Lamb – only once a week.
Beef – only once every 10–14 days.
Fish – once or twice a week.
Take pulses and whole grains for protein requirement –

including soya, haricot, aduki and kidney beans, lentils, chickpeas or Tofu – in at least three meals per week.

At least two meals per week should consist of brown rice and vegetables and bean sprouts only.

Potatoes, brown rice, barley, millet or millet and potato.

Pumpkin.

Any fruit, except bananas and oranges.

Beverages:

China or Earl Grey tea without milk or sugar.

Herb teas – drink one cup of sage tea per day. Elderflower tea is good. Try an infusion of elderflower and peppermint with a sprinkling of hops for flavour.

Drink one or two cups of fresh carrot juice per day.

Dressings, oils and condiments:

Dress salads with Molkosan, olive oil or cider vinegar.

Use garlic frequently in cooking and dressings.

Use only safflower, sunflower or olive oil, sparingly.

Use ample herbs, especially sage.

Use Herbamare salt.

Foods to be avoided:

Chocolate, cheese, eggs, cow's milk, butter, yoghurt, processed foods, white flour, white sugar, cakes, biscuits, bread, citrus fruits, coffee, white flour products, red wine, excess alcohol, malt vinegar, smoked or pickled foods, yeast extracts, animal fats. Smoking is prohibited.

Supplements:

Soya, lecithin and riboflavin (vitamin B2) are especially beneficial. A daily dose of 50,000 IU of vitamin A is often used in psoriasis therapy. The use of oil of evening primrose is also advisable.

In this diet I have been careful to avoid any foods which may act as an allergen to psoriasis sufferers, as I regard this as a distinctly possible cause of the condition. This approach cannot eliminate all possibilities, because the food we eat or the water we drink are not the only factors, pollution of air and environment are also relevant. In my book *Nature's Gift of Food* I have given detailed examples of the suitability of low protein or high carbohydrate diets and such knowledge is important for a successful approach to psoriasis. High protein is thought to aggravate the condition and therefore pork in any shape or form is not allowed. I must emphasise the use of carbohydrates and already I hear worried voices that this will cause an increase in weight. Nothing is further from the truth, because the diet is so well worked out that it will not cause weight gain. The diet is also aimed at being toxin-free, and in order to gain success as quickly as possible, I would further recommend that, wherever possible, organically-grown food should be used. If there are indications of a slight weight gain, take three or four Kelpasan tablets with a glass of hot water first thing in the morning. This is an excellent prevention for food poisoning or food toxicity.

As usual, efficient digestion and absorption are of great importance and so the food pattern must be right. If constipation is a chronic problem, I advise patients to follow Dr Vogel's Rasayana Programme, or 'Spring Cleansing Course'. Together with the diet I have often found this a good foundation for a psoriasis programme. Cleansing should be comprehensive, beginning with the liver, gallbladder, kidneys, and bloodstream. Sometimes a raw food diet, combined with zinc and essential fatty acids and herbs, like burdock, stinging nettle, dandelions, and skull cap, is of great help.

Let me remind you again that every effort should be made to control this condition, because psoriasis can spread at a most alarming rate, often thought to be even faster than cancer. It is quite amazing that statistics point to a psoriasis incidence as high as two to three per cent. The naturopathic view, that has been held for some time, is that the cause of psoriasis lies in a thinning of the small intestinal walls which allows poisons to enter into the circulatory system, and therefore the lymphatic system, manifesting itself in irritations on the skin. Whatever the cause, the sooner the problem is recognised and action is taken, the better for the patient.

I have seen great improvements in patients who decided on a course of fasting, and also in some patients who used bicarbonate of soda or Epsom salts in the bath water. The use of sulphur as a major detoxifying agent, together with vitamin B_6 is recommended. I also think that vitamin A is necessary, although it should not be taken indiscriminately because, in some psoriatic patients there are indications of liver involvement. The liver may be allergic to certain foods, or sometimes we just demand too much from this ever-industrious organ. It is like a well-run laboratory which never stops – it cleans 1,200 pints of blood every twenty-four hours – and it performs less effectively if there is too much vitamin A.

I observed the effects of a vitamin A surplus at close hand during a period of training with Dr Vogel in Switzerland. There we often spent long days working in the hot mountain sunshine. Black or brown patches appeared on the skin and nails of some of the workers indicating that, because of the strong sunshine, too much vitamin A was being absorbed. This is a note of caution to those *psoriasis* sufferers who are convinced that sunray treatment improves their skin condition.

Vitamin A ensures the healthy growth and repair of cells in all parts of the body, from the eyes to the intestines. It is not only an important thymus gland nutrient, but helps the entire immune system. Sufficient vitamin A is also required to maintain the defensive mucous membranes of the lungs, throat, nose and mouth so that pollutants and germs can be trapped and excreted. In a similar way, its cell-protection capabilities ensure smooth scalp and skin, our double organ of protection and secretion. Vitamin A is required for vision, as it keeps the eyes from drying out and forms part of the light-sensitive pigments of the eye. It is involved in the production of blood and the formation of bones and teeth.

Vitamin D is the sunshine vitamin because it is produced in the body in response to the action of sunlight on our skin. Because vitamin D is so important for the absorption of calcium and the use of phosphorus to form healthy bones and teeth, people who feel they do not get enough sunlight often choose to supplement their diet with vitamin D. Calcium and phosphorus are also vital for the health of the nervous system and normal blood-clotting. Nature's Best combine a natural form of vitamin D with vitamin A, which helps the body utilise it to its best advantage.

Although sunrays may have a healing effect on psoriasis patches, it is important that a sun filter cream is used. An excellent example is the P20 Sunfilter cream manufactured by the German company Riemann & Co. This product was tested for the Institute of Applied Skin Physiology by Karlheinz Schrader Laboratories in Holzminden, West Germany.

When visiting the beach, bathing in sea water and wading through seaweed is also therapeutic. The natural minerals in seaweed, such as sodium, potassium, iron and magnesium, encourage a better balance. This can also be achieved by mud baths, hot and cold fomentations, or castor oil fomentations.

Urticalcin is a homoeopathic remedy containing stinging nettle and will help to improve the skin condition of a psoriatic patient. Dabbing the affected parts with Molkosan will ease the inflammation. Usually Hepar Sulf 3x together with Rhus Tox 4x, is also helpful, and if the condition is very persistent I would recommend high potencies of Formic Acid 3x, together with graphite powder.

Fortunately psoriasis is not contagious, which means that even perspiration cannot cause it to spread, although this doesn't mean that the problem should be ignored. A raw food diet has always proved very successful and many of my patients believe that this was the decisive factor in the improvement of their condition. For the best results it is advisable to fast for a few days, and then follow this with a period when raw fruit and vegetables only are eaten. Because of the dietary link, essential fatty acids are of great importance and I would strongly recommend that three or four capsules of evening primrose oil are taken every night before going to bed.

You may be dazzled with all the treatment options open to you. I appreciate that it may not be easy to find the right treatment, but you will agree that the reward of a clear skin would be more than worth the effort. I remember a young nurse who was unable to accept her skin condition and refused to give up, going from one practitioner to another in her search for a cure. I suggested a programme that included dietary advice, vitamin supplements, evening primrose oil, herbal teas, and a few homoeopathic remedies, and asked her if she was prepared to follow my advice. Although she was initially sceptical, she agreed to follow my recommendations and was eventually rewarded with success. She was particularly pleased to reflect that her recovery was largely the result of her own perseverance: we may be dealing with a very stubborn disease, but it is not incurable.

For the last time I would remind you that skin diseases are an outward symptom of what is going on inside the body. Having read this book, you now realise that the causes of skin diseases may differ greatly, but an answer can always be found, if only we do not give up hope and continue to search for a solution. Whether the treatment is orthodox or complementary, bear in mind Calvin Coolidge's advice, 'Persistance and determination alone are potent factors'.

Worldwide it is thought that there are about eighteen million people who suffer from psoriasis, which is more than one in fifty. From experience I can promise you that all forms of psoriasis will improve when a well-balanced diet and herbal or homoeopathic remedies are used. *Psoriasis annularis*, for example, requires a different approach than

Psoriasis pulmaris. The latter usually affects the palms of the hands and the soles of the feet, and requires mainly external treatment. *Psoriasis diffusa* manifests itself in large lesions, whereas the lesions in *Psoriasis punctate* consist of minute papillae. *Psoriasis universalis* is possibly the most common form of this disease and produces lesions all over the body.

Sometimes, for a very persistent psoriatic condition, it may be necessary to apply acupuncture treatment. Such treatment must encompass the acupuncture law of the five elements, in which case it will result in an adrenal cortoid action or affect the thyroid and the endocrines. Acupuncture can be of tremendous value in certain cases of psoriasis, as can biomagnetic treatment. Copper needles should be used on the large patches and treatment should take place at regular intervals. Even I am sometimes still surprised when I see how quickly scabs and scales disappear after acupuncture treatment.

Hopefully I have by now managed to convince the psoriasis patient that the problem is not hopeless and that there are endless treatment combinations. Have faith in your practitioner, co-operate and the desired results will come. At heart I will always remain an old-fashioned naturopath and, as such, I remind you of the saying that 'Beauty comes from within'; cherish your inner health and a beautiful skin will be the result.

Bibliography

Harry Benjamin, *Everybody's Guide to Nature Cure*, Thorsons Publishing, Wellingborough, UK.

Bircher Benner, *Huidziekten*, De Driehoek, Amsterdam, The Netherlands.

Kitty Campion, *Handbook of Herbal Health*, Sphere Books Limited, London.

Leon Chaitow, *Skin Troubles*, Thorsons Publishing Group, Rochester, Vermont, USA.

Harry Clements, *Psoriasis*, Grafton Books, Harper Collins Publishers, London, UK.

Dr Carolyn Dean, *When You Can't Reach the Doctor*, Perfect Pitch Editions, W. Toronto, Canada.

Ilse Dorran, *De Natuur Uw Arts*, La Riviere en Voorhoeve, Kampen, The Netherlands.

Dorothy Hall, *The Natural Health Book*, Thomas Nelson Australia, Melbourne, Victoria.

Leonard Mervyn, *Complete Guide to Vitamins and Minerals*, Thorsons Publishing, Wellingborough, UK.

Christine Orton, *Eczema Relief*, Harper Collins Publishers, London, UK.

Dr A. Vogel, *Swiss Nature Doctor*, A. Vogel Verlag, Teufen, Switzerland.

Stella Weller, *Super Healthy Hair, Skin and Nails*, Harper Collins Publishers, London, UK.

Index

126